Music Therapy in Dementia Care

of related interest

Music Therapy and Neurological Rehabilitation
Performing Health
Edited by David Aldridge
ISBN 1 84310 302 8

Health, the Individual, and Integrated Medicine
Revisiting an Aesthetic of Health Care
David Aldridge
ISBN 1 84310 232 3

Case Study Designs in Music Therapy
Edited by David Aldridge
ISBN 184310 140 8

Music Therapy Research and Practice in Medicine
From Out of the Silence
David Aldridge
ISBN 1 85302 296 9

Music Therapy in Palliative Care
New Voices
Edited by David Aldridge
ISBN 1 85302 739 1

Music Therapy in Context
Music, Meaning and Relationship
Mercedes Pavlicevic
ISBN 1 85302 434 1

Spirituality, Healing and Medicine
Return to the Silence
David Aldridge
ISBN 1 85302 554 2

Suicide
The Tragedy of Hopelessness
David Aldridge
ISBN 1 85302 444 9

Music Therapy in Dementia Care

More New Voices

Edited by

David Aldridge

Jessica Kingsley Publishers
London and Philadelphia

First published in the United Kingdom in 2000
by Jessica Kingsley Publishers
116 Pentonville Road
London N1 9JB, UK
and
400 Market Street, Suite 400
Philadelphia, PA 19106, USA

www.jkp.com

Copyright © Jessica Kingsley Publishers 2000
Printed digitally since 2002

Library of Congress Cataloging in Publication Data
A CIP catalog record for this book is available from the Library of Congress

British Library Cataloguing in Publication Data
A CIP catalogue record for this book is available from the British Library

ISBN-13: 978 1 85302 776 5
ISBN-10: 1 85302 776 6

Contents

This book is dedicated to Konrad Schily

Angels' Wings

Exquisite precision of human soul.
Arrival.
Sweet explosion of new born.
We cherish softness.
Plumpness of early skin.
Yet before night is day we become youth.
Faltering.

Knowledge or innocence.
Which is worse?
Time called before time lived or wisdom silenced?
Tears flow and angels' wings flutter.
Both youth and age pass fleetingly.

Gillian Hogan

CHAPTER I

Overture: It's Not What You Do But the Way that You Do It

David Aldridge

While writing this introduction the words to an old song were running through my head. I was looking for a likely caption to sum up what I was trying to say and found myself singing 'It's not what you do but the way that you do it. It's not what you say but the way that you say it'. And, like all responsible authors of scientific essays, and certainly as a research supervisor and mentor who hammers home the necessity of quoting sources, I tried to remember from where the song came. But could I remember for the life of me? How frustrating the sense of failing memory. Yet the melody lingers on. And that is the message of this book. While the memory of the source fails, the music lingers on. When we sing, the words, emotions and situations can be re-called. Maybe there is something to do with the very word that we use to describe memory; it is a sense of recall, as if there is a voice that calls the memory back. When those memories return, they are also re-collected. We put them together to make sense of them. Sense is made, it is an activity, like making music. We shall also see that the same goes for story-telling. Old stories, like old songs, are called forth from then to now and woven together as the fabric of reality.

There is an important element to music that carries over to speech. If I want to tell you something, then I can give you the information by telling you the content. This works very well for arranging a meeting: 'Eight o'clock on Friday night under the bus station clock'. Ah, the memories. But if I want to tell you something important, like 'I miss you', then it is not only the words that are important, but also the way in which the words are said that convey the intent, as every lover will know. With words we can lie: the expression gives the clue to how what is said is to be understood. It is not what you say, but the way that you say it; and that is where the music comes into communication.

When we cannot remember by ourselves, then we require assistance. We all have experiences of talking about old times with a friend and how each of us brings varying strands of recollection that weave together the tapestry of memory. This is clearly demonstrated in Chapter 3 by the writer Trisha Kotai-Ewers.To enable us to weave this magic carpet upon which memories ride, music therapists have been honing their varying skills, as the following chapters will illustrate. These are musical skills, in knowing what music will cue a memory trace, and relationship skills, in knowing how to calm or arouse us such that the conditions for the cue are set. I emphasize both sets of skills here as music therapists use music 'receptively', that is, playing chosen music to another person in a therapeutic way, and 'actively', in that music therapy can have a performative component where both therapist and patient make music together. Chapter 7 by Gudrun Aldridge, Chapter 8 by Fraser Simpson and Chapter 9 by Susan Weber remind us of this mutuality. Both forms of activity, receptive listening or making music together, require the essentials of relationship and knowledge.

While music is being championed as an important intervention in various settings for those advanced in years, music therapy is simply not a matter of putting a compact disc in the hi-fi system. Throughout the years, I have been asked for a suitable repertoire for elderly people. The question usually goes: 'My mum is 80, living alone, and I want to buy her some compact discs to play at home so that she isn't so lonely. What would you prescribe?' The answer that invariably follows is:

> Well, first we cannot prescribe music like medication. But you can ask her what she likes, or probably over the years, being your mother you have probably got to know her well (like a mother, really), then you know what she likes. Secondly, compact discs are no substitute for companionship. They share the first four letters, but that is all. Loneliness is not cured by music and as every young lover knows, music probably makes loneliness deliciously worse.

So the challenge is not to stick another record on the record machine but to sing to your mother. By singing with another person, we have to adjust our singing to the way in which they react and we shall see this in Chapter 4 by Alicia Ann Clair and Chapter 10 by Connie Tomaino. And there lie the music therapy skills; in musical judgement of the appropriate repertoire, knowing when to respond and when to pull back, as every bar-pianist will tell you.

Hand–ear co-ordination

We know from our work with children that music therapy facilitates and enables communication. Indeed, we know that there is an innate musicality to human communication. I have taken this a step further and suggested that the process of living is performative, that we are polyrhythmic, symphonic beings improvised in the moment. This is to emphasize 'I perform therefore I am', rather than the Cartesian 'I think therefore I am'.

Working with developmentally delayed children we found that thinking, and the development of cognitive abilities, were developed out of musical abilities; careful listening in a relationship, joint attention and hand and eye co-ordination were encouraged by musical playing. Potentials emerge and these demand the participation of another. What appears to be important is the co-ordination of sensory modes intra-individually and inter-individually (Aldridge 1996). Just as the baby co-ordinates hand and mouth, then we see the infant also co-ordinating hands and eyes, hands and ears. Hands, eyes, ears, mouth, feet, all speak of an inherent ability of the body to combine its efforts to co-ordinate with itself and with others in an ecology of the senses. Working with developmentally challenged children, we find that handicap is itself disabled by music. This is not a 'Mozart' effect, it is a 'Joe Bloggs' effect. By playing music we achieve our own individual genius, but in the company of another. If genius emerges, then it is an accompanied geniality. Here individuals achieve themselves but in co-operation with another. Personal identities are performed and they are themselves works of 'street' art demanding an audience. We are performers performing our roles together in the mutual dances of relationship, songs of comradeship and anthems of solidarity.

What is central to these performances is that they occur now. There is a subjective present that is recognized, and the relationship facilitates the presence of the present. The now of mammalian movement has an estimated duration. Music is the scaffolding of time in which the present is constructed. The construction in time, that we call now, when extended is the stuff of short-term memory and the basis of cognition. That is how music therapy works: it offers a form for events that develops as memory. Thus musical playing, and communication, is prior to cognition.

If this happens for children then the same process can occur at the end of life. With the problems of elderly people exhibiting dementia their lives are severely curtailed cognitively. The tragedy of Alzheimer's disease is that all the sufferers, while retaining perception, lose their ability to perform. They lose their 'now' of existence, becoming dislocated in space and disoriented in time. How is it possible to perform a 'self' that is coherent in these circumstances? Such a question begins to be answered within the pages of this book where practitioners demonstrate how the creative act, in relationship, allows people to perform identities that are not stigmatized where the self can be expressed in the breadth of its capacities. Central to this expression is an awareness of now and the ability to perform in the present. It is music that offers this form for the present as well as calling to the past. The past is called forth into the present and realized anew. These memories too are composed; they may lack accuracy but their potency remains the same. They have their themes and their feelings and while being mediated by the brain, may originate in our feet.

In Chapter 2, Melissa Brotons gives us an account of how varying music therapy practitioners and theorists have attempted to understand how they can help those suffering with dementia, particularly the Alzheimer's type. In Chapters 5 and 6, Annemiek Vink, who works in the Netherlands, writes how such understandings are being brought into the field of geriatric practice specifically for the management of agitation, and how music therapists carry out their work in psychogeriatry.

Time and space

To act in the world we need the vital coordinates of time and space. We exist in the now and here. While we consider chronological time as important for what we do in terms of co-ordination, it is the idea of time as kairos that is significant. If chronos is time as measured, kairos is time considered as the right or opportune moment. It contains elements of appropriateness and purpose. Inherent within the term is the concept of decisiveness; there is tension within the moment that calls for a decision. In addition, there is also the expectation that a purpose will be accomplished. While musicians may well play according to a measured time, it is the decisiveness of playing that gives music its rhythm. Rhythm demands intention. Furthermore, the very stuff of improvised playing together is a series of purposive decisions made in the moment that must be acted upon. Kairos reigns where creative purposes are to be achieved.

Patients suffering with a dementia are prisoners of mechanical time. They have not a chronic illness but a kairotic illness (Aldridge 1996). The difficulty lies in making decisions in the moment and acting upon them. If motivation is a problem for elderly people suffering with dementia, it is precisely that initiation cannot take place; the act cannot be brought into being and therefore purposes remain uncompleted. In this way, dementia is not something that makes sense, it is something that no longer makes time. While sufferers are in time, as chronological events among the rest of the world and its myriad of happenings, they are no longer of time. This is where our musical understanding of time will bring a significant perspective to bear in the discovery of what it is to be demented. Mentation is a kairotic process not solely understandable in its chronology. De-mentation is the discoupling in kairotic time of physiological events.

Actions, however, are not restricted to time; they occur in space. We co-ordinate the movement of our limbs to particular places. Movements have an intention that is localized eventually. To dance you have to move your feet in time and know where to put them. The same goes for playing music. We have in some ways become overbalanced in our emphasis on the brain. While it is undeniably necessary, and it is the plaques of Alzheimer's disease in the brain that are interfering with function, maybe it is in our body where memories are stored. It is our feet that know how to dance, just as our fingers remember how to play and our hearts remember how to love. If we try thinking about how to ride a bicycle then cognition is of little help. Getting on the bicycle and riding it, the essential bodily activity, is that which achieves the performance. Thus, playing music, dancing, moving, telling, these activities are prior in the invocation of memory as the calling forth of a performed identity.

The body has perhaps been neglected in communication studies as we emphasize language, yet it is gesture that is pre-verbal and promotes cognition. Posture, movement and prosodics in relationship provide the bases for communication. Through the medium of an active performed body, health is expressed and maintained. Here it is bodily form that guides communication and by which the other may be understood. It has an ambiguous content and it is social. Language provides a specific content and it is cultural. We know that someone is suffering by their appearance; what the specific nature of that suffering is they need to tell us. We know someone is happy by what they do; what makes them so happy, they need to tell us. In addition, by moving as if we were happy, we may promote happiness. By moving as if we were sad, we may promote sadness. Thus the body, and a moved body at that, is central to a life among others.

A performed identity and a constructed narrative

There is a profound level of understanding that lies beyond, or before, verbal communication. Underlying the concept of a performed identity is the notion that we 'do' who we are. We perform our very selves in the world as activities. This is as basic as our physiology and provides the ground of immunology, a performance of the self to maintain its identity. Over and above this, we have the performance of a personality, not separate from the body, for which the body serves as an interface to the social world. We also perform that self among other performers, we have a social world in which we 'do' our lives with others. This is the social self that is recognized and acknowledged by our friends, lovers and colleagues. This performed identity is not solely dependent upon language but is composed rather like a piece of jazz. We are improvised each day to meet the contingencies of that day. And improvised with others, who may prove to be the very contingencies that day has to offer.

We perform our identities and they have to have form for communication to occur. Such form is like musical form. Language provides the content for those per-form-ances. Thus we need an authored identity to express the distress in a coherent way with others to generate intelligible accounts (Csordas 1983). We have a network of coherent symbols as performed narratives. If language fails then the opportunity for us to accord our form, as selves, with others, appears to fail.

Narratives are constructed and interpreted. They lend meaning to what happens in daily life. We all have our biographies. What happens to our bodies is related to our identities as persons. These narratives are not simply personal stories, but sagas negotiated in the contexts of our intimate relationships. These understandings are also constructed within a cultural context that lend legitimacy to those narratives. Thus meanings are nested within a hierarchy of contexts. The same process applies to the history of our bodies, to the biography of our selves, to the narratives used by clinicians, or to the tales told by the elders of a tribe (Aldridge 2000).

Patients and their family have a story about the problems they face. And this story has to be told. It is in the telling that we understand what needs are. It is also in this act of telling that we have the opportunity to express ourselves. The expression of our needs is a performative activity. Patients' narratives about their illness do not always point out the meaning directly, but demonstrate meaning by recreating pattern in metaphorical shape or form in the telling that is interpreted within relationship. Symptoms in an illness narrative are a symbolic communication as they are told and confessed. Symptoms are signs that have to be observed and interpreted in their performance. We know that many elderly people visit their general practitioner expressing pain and expecting a physical examination. Very few say directly that it is painful being lonely and that they are rarely touched. In a culture where it is not allowed to express such emotional needs of suffering and touch directly, then the narrative becomes a medical story of pain. Suffering is embodied as pain. While we may temporarily relieve pain with analgesics, our task is also to understand, and thereby relieve, suffering. In this way the ecology of ideas, that some call knowledge, is explicated within the body as a correspondence between mental representations and the material world. The setting in which we express ourselves will have an influence upon what we express. An extension of this will be that we, as caregivers, are open to the expression of other narratives. Creative arts therapists then will be only too aware of the possibilities of symbolic communication. We are the setting that narratives may be creatively expressed as we shall read in Chapter 3 by Trisha Kotai-Ewers and Chapter 10 by Connie Tomaino.

Meanings are linked to actions, and those actions have consequences that are performed. What our patients think about the causes of their illnesses will influence what they do in terms of treatment, which in turn will influence what they do in the future. As practitioners, we lend meaning to the events that are related to us by our patients, weaving them into the fabric of our treatment strategies. We must learn to understand each other's language for expressing and resolving distress, and act consequently. These expressions are non-verbal and predicated upon bodily expressions, that can be seen in movement; or vocal, that are sung; or visual, that are painted. In this way the creative arts offer not only contexts for expression, but also contexts for resolution, congruent to the mode in which patients choose to perform themselves.

For verbally inarticulate people, this has an important ramification as they are offered understanding and the potential for resolution of their distress. For elderly people suffering with dementia, although verbal communication fails, we can offer contexts of expression and understanding where gesture, movement and vocalization make communicative sense.

For those struggling with verbal articulation, the structuring of narratives offers a meaningful context in which expression can occur. Remembering a story offers an overarching framework that links events together. This is reflected in the concept of re-collection. We collect the episodes and events of our memories together again. We shall see later that when a piece of favourite music is played, there is a cascade of memories from an initial musical prompting, even if we cannot remember the name of the composer or lyricist. As individuals we are stories, we are composed and those compositions remain. In a series of studies by Pennebaker (Dienstfrey 1999), writing as disclosure of distressing experiences has clear health-care benefits.

Health as performance in a praxis aesthetic

Performed health is dependent upon a variety of negotiated meanings, and how those meanings are transcended. As human beings we continue to develop. Body and self are narrative constructions, stories that are related to intimates at chosen moments. Meanings are linked to actions, and those actions have consequences that are performed. The maintenance and promotion of health, or becoming healthy, is an activity. As such it will be expressed bodily, a praxis aesthetic.

The social is incorporated, literally 'in the body', and that incorporation is transcended through changes in consciousness, which become themselves incarnate. Through the body we have articulations of distress and health. While health may be concerned with the relief of distress, and can also be performed for its own sake, sickness is a separate phenomenon. It is possible to have a disease but not be distressed. Indeed, it is possible to be dying and not be distressed. Yet for those who are described as being demented, there is a schism between the social and the body. When communication fails, we literally 'fall out' with other people, we fall out of relationship. This is evident in the social difficulties that demented people have: they fail to connect to the rhythms of daily life, to other people and within themselves. We lose our consciousness when connections fail and these are literally organic in the context of dementia and the implications are far-reaching when our body falls out with our 'self'. We have lost an inherent ecology.

If we take my earlier metaphor of composition, when bodily function fails, then we are literally de-composed. Yet as human beings we know that, despite our physical failings, something remains within us. There is a self that responds. Despite all that medical science will have to offer us regarding the decomposition of the physical body, it is the composition of the self that we must address in our therapeutic endeavours. It is to the psychological and humanistic sciences that we must direct our attention if we are to gain the knowledge necessary that will aid us in working with those who come to us for help. Indeed, it is our memories of the other that helps the dementia sufferer compose his or her self. In relationship we foster a return to those ecological connections. And it is music that forms the basis of relationship through rhythm and timbre (Aldridge 1996).

The coherent body and the subjective now

The body becomes an interface for the expression of identity that is personal and social. In a metaphysical tradition, the human being is considered as a self-contained consciousness, *homo clausus*, yet Smith (1999) argues for an alternative model, *homo aperti*, the idea that human beings gain identity through participation in social groups. My argument, so far, is that this identity is performed. Both the personal and the social are necessary. Bodies express themselves at the interface of the personal and the social. Using the body communicates to others. Using the body achieves perception of the environment, and that includes those with whom we live. But the performance of the body requires a biological system that is intact, a system that remains coherent over time. Memory is the coherence of events in time. When memory fails then a sequence of events lose their coherence. Not only that, if we fail to respond to events that demand a return performance, we are perceived as unresponsive. And the coherence of events is a rudimentary narrative. Our perception of self is dependent upon coherence in time.

I have used earlier the concept of human being as being like a piece of improvised music. For the piece to work as music it has to maintain coherence. We could just as well take a raga form where a theme is improvised to its limits, the tension lying in the variation and its relationship to the original theme. To achieve coherence we have to engage in a form that exists in time. A piece of music achieves coherence in its maintenance of form. Exactly so with our personal form in social life. If we lose time, then we lose our sense of coherence, and we lose our cognitive abilities too. Just as children gain cognitive abilities with their increasing ability to hold events together coherently in time, then we see the reverse process in the performance of the demented – demented being literally without mental form. This may occur as a performance difficulty through the loss of connections. Within us, there is still a self, with its continuing story that has a developmental need. How is that story then to be expressed? How does the narrative continue such that the saga is told to its end? To do this we need to reconnect. As we see in recovering coma patients, it is the connection of existing capacities in a context of joint attention that leads to an improvement in consciousness (Aldridge

1990, 1996). With elderly patients who are demented, therapy must be directed to connecting what intrinsic abilities remain. While these may not be verbal there are other possibilities of sound and movement.

Understanding each other

Our stories are our identities. How we relate them to each other constructively, so that we mutually understand each other, is the basis of communication. What we do, or persuade others to do, as a consequence of those communicated stories is an exercise of power. How narratives are interpreted is important for understanding the ensuing possibilities of treatment. If a person is seen as being illegitimate in her demands for treatment then she may be seen as a social case not needing medical help, and this is critical at a time of stretched medical resources. If a person is seen as being aggressive in his demands by the way in which he expresses himself then he may be sedated rather than change the setting in which he finds himself. This process of problem resolution has consequences for the continuing narration of a patient biography that becomes dislocated from a healthy personal biography. If we become dislocated from our personal biographies then we suffer. Either we are labelled as deviant and become stigmatized, or we become isolated.

In elderly people who become demented, we see individuals dislocated from their biographies socially, by entering into caring institutions, and personally. Memory fails, and with it self fails to achieve a performance in daily life that integrates varying faculties. The very 'I' that is myself fails to perform the 'me' that we all know. Thus the interface that is self in performance loses its narrative form. Fortunately, the fundamental basis of communication on which that performance is based, our inherent musicality, remains. In the following chapters we shall see how skilled practitioners invoke what is still there. The 'I' finds its 'me'. All is not lost. There is hope and with that hope then healing.

Anecdotes as scientific stories

> The point of these therapies is not so much to cure the individual as to develop forms of viable meaning. (Gergen 1997, p.26)

Throughout this book the reader will find a series of stories. The stories that patients tell. The stories that therapists tell. These are the very stuff of clinical life and bring important material for understanding our way forward with the people who come to us for help. My argument is that not only is the very stuff of life performed but that science, the gaining and transmission of knowledge, is structured too as a narrative. By trying to confine us to restricted narrative forms, the experimental procedure, then we are being submitted to censure. This is a political act that seeks to limit the expression of what we know, the form that we know it and the forms that we can express it. Therefore I have asked my colleagues in this book to express themselves in the forms that they find most comfortable to express what they want to convey. There are powerful stories here about human suffering and its relief that are vital for us to understand in the current climate of health care. If we fail to heed them, it is not because of the failure of their expression, it is because those that are charged with hearing have deafened themselves to the voices of what is being proclaimed.

Complementary medical approaches are often dismissed as relying upon anecdotal material, as if stories are unreliable. My argument is that stories are reliable and rich in information. Indeed, it is a complaint made by patients of modern medical practitioners that they are not allowed to tell their own stories and a reason given why they turn to alternative medical practitioners who give them time to explain their problem in their own terms. While we as medical scientists may try to dismiss the anecdote, we rely upon it when we wish to explain particular cases to our colleagues away from the conference podium (Aldridge 1996; R. Miller 1998). Even in scientific medicine, it has been the single case report that has been necessary to alert practitioners to the negative side-effects of current treatment (Aldridge 1992).

While anecdotes may be considered as bad science, they are the everyday stuff of clinical practice. People tell us their stories and expect to be heard. Stories have a structure and are told in a style that informs us too. It is not solely the content of a story, it is how it is told that convinces us of its validity. While questionnaires gather information about populations, and view the world from the perspective of the researcher, it is talking together that provides the condition for patients to generate their meaningful story. The relationship is the context for the story and patients' stories may change according to the conditions in which they are related. Anecdotes are the very stuff of social life and the fabric of communication in the healing encounter.

When people come to their practitioners they are asking about what will become of them. What will their future be like? Will there be a change? Some practitioners make a prognosis based on the interview that they have had with the patient. Sometimes this will be the dreaded answer to the question

'How long do I have to live?' But, with each interview there is the question of when healing will take place. What can be expected in the near future and is there any hope of a cure? The story of what happens is, in part, a clinical history. It is also no less than the narration of destiny, the unfolding of a person's life purpose (Larner 1998).

Change is concerned with how the future meets the past and how we make sense of such a transition. In narratives there is the possibility to open up to something new. This is where the potential for healing takes place and where we can introduce hope, the moment that transcends what has gone before. Narratives bring a coherence and order to life stories. Stories make sense. As we read earlier, the subjective now has to be performed, and this can be assisted, recalled and recollected. The past is called into the present, the self is composed anew, and we are no longer a series of isolated events divorced from meaning but coherent stories that are ever unfolding.

When we consider narratives about the future then we construct possible life courses based upon our own agency. Of course we have to consider the realities of disability, but those realities may differ according to the setting in which we find ourselves. The variance of my disability to perform will be contingent upon those with whom I interact. Hope is what lifts me out of the moment of my disability to a new possibility. In this way, the person with whom I am is also the source of my potential and possibility, the source of my hope. Thus the therapeutic relationship bears a responsibility for offering alternative chances for performance.

Usually, we choose the people with whom our narrative will be told in the future. We choose the people who will influence that narrative. Agency in this sense is the ability to shift between the principles under which life is lived and the potential discourses that will be used to describe such a life. This does not mean that demented people will escape dementia. But the narrative of disability that we perform, how our abilities are performed, with whom we are able and how those abilities are remembered, is important. Hope lies in the ability to perform such a narrative. Distress lies in the disability to perform our life's story further.

Incidence and prevalence

Alzheimer's disease is and will become an enormous public health problem. Interventions that could delay disease onset even modestly would have a major public health impact. In 1997, the numbers of individuals in the United States with Alzheimer's disease was estimated at 2.32 million (range:

1.09 million to 4.58 million); of these individuals, 68 per cent were female. The numbers of newly diagnosed cases that can be expected over the next 50 years were estimated from a model that used age-specific incidence rates summarized from several epidemiological studies and it is projected that the prevalence will nearly quadruple in the next 50 years, by which time approximately 1 in 45 Americans will be afflicted with the disease (Brookmeyer, Gray and Kawas 1998).

The prevalence of dementia in subjects 65 years and older in North America is approximately 6–10 per cent, with Alzheimer's disease (AD) accounting for two-thirds of these cases (Hendrie 1998). If milder cases are included, the prevalence rates double. While a genetic basis for Alzheimer's disease has been identified, the search for non-genetic risk factors has been less conclusive. Only age and family history of dementia are consistently associated with AD in all studies.

Research approaches to new treatments

Until the mid 1980s, psychotherapy and counselling techniques had rarely been used with people with dementia. However, the change in emphasis within dementia care towards a person-centred approach, and often non-pharmacological approach, has meant that there is a growing clinical interest in their use (Beck 1998; Bender and Cheston 1997; Bonder 1994; Cheston 1998; Johnson, Lahey and Shore 1992; Richarz 1997). This has also meant an increase in studies using creative arts therapies (Bonder 1994; Harlan 1993; Johnson et al. 1992; Kamar 1997; Mango 1992) and overviews of music therapy as a treatment approach to Alzheimer's disease have already been written (Aldridge and Brandt 1991; Brotons, Koger and Pickett-Cooper 1997; Smeijsters 1997) as Melissa Brotons writes in Chapter 2. What music therapy offers is an improvement in communication skills for sufferer and spousal caregiver, and possibilities for managing the disruption and agitation ensuing in the later stages of disease.

Individuals with Alzheimer's disease often experience depression, anger and other psychological symptoms. Various forms of psychotherapy have been attempted with these individuals, including insight-oriented therapy and less verbal therapies such as music therapy and art therapy. Although there are few data-based outcome studies that support the effectiveness of these interventions, case studies and descriptive information suggest that they can be helpful in alleviating negative emotions and minimizing problematic behaviours (Bonder 1994).

Although there is a developing clinical literature on intervention techniques drawn from all the main psychotherapeutic approaches, there has been little research into the effectiveness of this work and such research as does exist often uses methodologies that are inappropriate for such an early stage of clinical development. While some authors (Cheston 1998) argue that clinical research should adopt case study or single-case designs, some researchers are also planning group designs for evaluating new clinical developments. My argument is for a broad spectrum of research designs that will satisfy differing needs. We know from experience that music therapy brings benefits to sufferers (see Table 1.1) and the challenge is to convert this knowledge into evidential studies.

Table 1.1 Clinical benefits of music therapy

	Maintenance and reattainment of skills
Communication skills: personal	encourages learning new material
	improves memory skills for a short period of time
Communication skills: social	motivates and encourages purposeful interaction
	promotes interaction within sessions
	fosters spontaneous behaviours in social situations
	advances spousal caregivers' communications skills
Behaviour management	reduces agitation and disruptive behaviour
	reduces anxiety

Annenmiek Vink in Chapter 6 focuses on the treatment of agitation in Alzheimer's disease using music therapy; her current work is in the administration of a controlled study in the Netherlands. The success of such a venture may have a profound effect upon the political acceptance of music therapy as a non-pharmacological treatment modality should the results be of significance. I am tentative about suggesting how strong the impact of such research trials will be as there is never any guarantee that such studies will be heeded. More importantly, if such a study discovers that a control musical condition is almost as effective as music therapy then there may be support for using 'music' in treatment settings but not necessarily music therapists. Given that music therapists are a professional group with their own pay scales, then while the argument for using musical initiatives may be strong, the argument for employing music specialists may be weak. Research, and its results, are rarely neutral in their effect.

However, as we see from the work of Gudrun Aldridge (Chapter 7), Fraser Simpson (Chapter 8), Susan Weber (Chapter 9) and Connie Tomaino (Chapter 10), qualitative understandings of how musical playing changes also offers profound insights into the relief of suffering. We simply cannot restrain our endeavours to one particular form of understanding. Differing research approaches will inform one another and the challenge is for us to co-ordinate our approaches such that the knowledge gained is pooled and shared. It is to such an end that this book is aimed.

Patients and their caregivers

In the absence of definitive treatments for Alzheimer's disease and related dementias, researchers in a variety of disciplines are developing psychosocial and behavioural intervention strategies to help patients and caregivers better manage and cope with the troublesome symptoms common in these conditions. These strategies include cognitive interventions, functional performance interventions, environmental interventions, integration of self-interventions, and pleasure-inducing interventions. Although we have seen that more research is needed to develop these strategies further and establish their best use, psychosocial and behavioural interventions hold great promise for improving the quality of life and well-being of dementia patients and their family caregivers (Beck 1998).

We know that people who are suffering do not suffer alone (Aldridge 1998a, 1999). It is in a primary care setting where dementia is recognized, and early recognition is important for initiating treatment interventions before a person becomes permanently or semi-permanently institutionalized and to minimize disability (Larson 1998). There is an increasing expectation that the community will care for its elderly infirm members, although this expectation is rarely met by financial resources that will support such caregiving, placing the caregivers under stress, while relieving a community budget in the short term.

Recent research on caregiver stress focuses extensively on its predictors and health consequences, especially for family members of persons with dementia. Gwyther and Strulowitz (1998) suggest four areas of caregiver stress research: caregiver health outcomes, differential impacts of social support, caregiving for family members with dementia, and balancing work and caregiving responsibilities.

In a study by Harris (1998), in-depth interviews with 30 sons actively involved in caring for a parent with dementia elicit the understanding of a son's caregiving experiences. Common themes that emerge from such narratives are a sense of duty, acceptance of the situation and having to take charge as well as issues regarding loss, a change in relationships with other brothers and sisters, the reversal of role from based on having to take charge and the necessity to develop coping strategies.

In another study of the psychological well-being of caregivers of demented elderly people (Pot, Deeg and Van Dyck 1997), three groups of caregivers were identified; those providing care for two years after baseline; those whose care-recipient died within the first year after baseline, and those whose care-recipient was institutionalized within the first year. All groups of caregivers showed a great amount of psychological distress compared to a general population sample, with an overall deterioration of psychological well-being. As the elderly patient declined, and the caregiving at home continued, then psychological distress increased. For caregivers whose demented care-recipient had died or was institutionalized in the first year after baseline, there was no deterioration. There is, then, a high level of psychological distress and deterioration in psychological well-being among informal caregivers of dementia patients and we may have to reconsider the personal and social costs of demented older people living on their own as long as possible if we are not able to release adequate resources to support the caregivers.

Part of this support will include sharing information and developing methods of counselling appropriate to caregivers. Increasing public awareness, coupled with the wider availability of drug therapies for some dementing conditions, means that carers are often informed of the diagnosis of dementia. However, it is unclear how much sufferers themselves are told about their diagnoses. In a study of how sufferers of dementia were given diagnostic information of 71 carers recruited through old age psychiatry services in East Anglia, half of the sufferers had learned their diagnosis more from their carers than their doctors (Heal and Husband 1998). The age of the sufferer was found to be related to whether or not doctors told them their diagnosis, which supports a suspicion that there is a prejudice among doctors regarding elderly patients and about what they can understand. Only 21 per cent of carers were given an opportunity to discuss the issues involved and younger carers were significantly more likely to feel that such an opportunity would have been useful. Most of the carers who had informed the sufferer said that the sufferer had wanted to know, or needed a meaningful explanation for their difficulties, rather than giving more practical legal or financial reasons. Carers who had not disclosed feared that diagnostic information would cause too much distress, or that the sufferers' cognitive impairments were too great an obstacle.

It's not what you say but the way that you say it

The process of 'informing' is a political act and demands the sharing of knowledge. While this is indeed a specialist medical task, the consequences of that task are explicated in a social nexus. Caregivers need to be informed that they can inform. As this chapter stated, it is not simply giving facts that are important, it is understanding how those facts will be understood in the context of relationship that is vital, or as in the following case, almost fatal.

An elderly man was recently informed after a series of tests that he had Parkinson's disease. His doctor was pleased that the tests had proved positive and at least now he, as physician, knew what the problem was. In his own mind, the man confused the diagnosis of Parkinson's with Alzheimer's disease, and on his way home from the surgery contemplated a life of disability and deterioration. His imaginings were of the worst scenario possible. He had his new medication that brought relief but his future was inevitably damaged and irretrievable. The past told him how he had been. From that past he predicted his future. A future that now was shattered. Hope had gone with the diagnosis that comforted his physician.

His wife had stayed at home not wanting to hear any bad news. As he entered the house, she knew from the expression on his face that something drastic had happened. He told her what his doctor had said and she too confused the diagnosis of Parkinson's with Alzheimer's disease into a misunderstanding of all the worst possible scenarios she had read about or seen on television. Her husband was surprised that she did not seem to react but sat calmly on the sofa. It was only when, after a while, this apparent calm became evidence of immobility and the right side of her mouth slumped, that he knew something was amiss. He rang for the emergency services and an ambulance arrived to rush her to hospital where she was treated for a stroke.

A simple intervention in the primary care setting, while costing time, might have drastically altered this scenario. It certainly exemplifies the importance of delivering information and the way that information is understood. Fortunately my parents are both well now and thanks to the Parkinsons' Self-Help group are optimally informed.

Modern medical care has helped undeniably in acute situations, while at the same time exhibiting a stunning disregard of what it is to be a human being and suffering. The doctor was secure in his understanding of the problem and for him it was a relief to make a diagnosis. What failed to be appreciated was the needs of the patient and how his understanding was not congruent with that of the practitioner. In the broadest sense of the term, knowledge as *diagnosis* is based not solely upon physiology but upon the deep needs of the patient and carers. Neither knowledge excludes the other; both can be reconciled. From such mutual knowledge, a *prognosis* can be made. Yet a prognosis, knowledge about the future, which surely is hope, is predicated upon what we do know. It is dependent upon relationship and the ensuing understanding, not with some statistical ideal but human contact. The diagnosis of a medical complaint is also a statement about personal identity and the stigma that may be attached to such an identity. Understandings are the loci of power whereby illness is explained and controlled. In the demand for caregiver information, such loci are shifting from the educated health professionals to increasingly better-educated caregivers as consumers.

Emotional context and ability

As we saw in the above example, it is important to consider the internal world of the sufferer. Bender and Cheston (1997) present a stage model of the subjective world of dementia sufferers drawing on ideas from both clinical and social psychology. The first stage involves feelings engendered by the process of dementia and includes four discrete states of anxiety, depression, grief and despair. The second stage of the model concerns the behaviours provoked by process of decline. Finally, a continuum of emotions is considered, where the ability of individuals with dementia to engage in emotional behaviour depends upon the extent of their cognitive impairment and the social context in which they are located. In another study (Vasterling *et al.* 1997) examining unawareness of social interaction and emotional control competency, both deficits are positively correlated with dementia severity.

As the disease progresses there is a degeneration of the ability to comprehend and express emotion that is linked with mental impairment (Benke, Bosch and Andree 1998). The creative arts therapies have based some of their interventions on the possibility for promoting emotional expression and retaining expressive abilities. As I suggested earlier, mental impairment may be one thing but the musical abilities that are the vehicles of expression remain.

Depression

Depression is a common disorder in elderly people (Forsell, Jorm and Winblad 1998). The rate of treatment of depression in very elderly people is low, exaggerated among dementia sufferers, and the course is chronic or relapsing in almost half of the cases. The interface between depression and dementia is complex and has been studied primarily in Alzheimer's disease (Aldridge 1993a) where depressive depression may be a risk factor for the expression of Alzheimer's disease in later life (Raskind 1998). A contributory factor to this depression is the patients' perceptions of their own deficits, although these may be ill founded (Tierney *et al.* 1996). Emotional context is an important factor and this will be linked to the way in which the patients see their current life situation and an understanding of what life holds in the near future.

Hope, where the past meets the future, is a major coping strategy for achieving the best out of a situation. Depression will work against this. Conversely, hope combats depression. It is here that we have to consider that hope may be contagious, not only do we have to promote hope in the patients but also in the caregivers. Just as depression runs in families, then hope too. But it has to be orchestrated.

Hearing impairment

If depression is a confounding factor in recognizing cognitive degeneration, then hearing impairment is another contributory factor. Central auditory test abnormalities may predict the onset of clinical dementia or cognitive decline. Hearing loss significantly lowered performance on the verbal parts of the Mini-Mental State Examination, a standard test for the presence of dementia (Gates *et al.* 1996). Central auditory dysfunction precedes senile dementia in a significant number of cases and may be an early marker for senile dementia. Gates *et al.* (1996) recommend that hearing tests should be included in the evaluation of persons older than 60 years and in those suspected of having cognitive dysfunction. If this is so then we may have to include this consideration in designs of research studies of music therapy as maybe the patients themselves are not actually hearing what is being played but responding to social contact and gesture. However, encouraging musical participation may foster residual hearing abilities and those abilities that the tests cannot measure. Returning to the developmentally challenged children, where hearing disability was ever present, it was the joint attention involved in making music that brought about an improvement in listening that appeared as an improvement in hearing. This is perhaps a feature of active music therapy that needs to be further investigated.

What happens

Most music therapists have concentrated on the pragmatic effects of music therapy. As we shall see, both practitioners and researchers alike are concerned with demonstrating the benefits of music therapy for dementia sufferers. However, how music therapy actually achieves its effects is relatively unresearched. My hypothesis is that music offers an alternative form for structuring time that fails in working memory. Just as developmentally delayed children achieve a working memory that enhances their cognitive ability, then the reverse process occurs in dementia sufferers.

While several components of working memory may be affected, not all aspects of the central executive mechanism are necessarily influenced (Collette *et al.* 1998). White and Murphy (1998) suggest that tone perception remains intact, but there is a progressive decline in working memory for auditory non-verbal information with advancing Alzheimer's disease. A similar decline was also noted on a task assessing working memory for auditory presented verbal information. This ties in with what we know about hearing impairment and again encourages a test of hearing capabilities before music therapy is used as a treatment modality but also suggests that music therapy may promote improved hearing.

Temporal coherence

I argued earlier that music therapy is indicated because it offers an external sense of temporal coherence that is failing in the patient. Ellis (1996) reports on the linguistic features and patterns of coherence in the discourse of mild and advanced Alzheimer's patients. As the disease progresses, the discourse of Alzheimer's patients becomes pre-grammatical in that it is vocabulary driven and reliant on meaning-based features of discourse rather than grammatically based features. Temporal coherence fails. Knott, Patterson and Hodges (1997), considering the short-term memory performance of patients with semantic dementia, suggest that impaired semantic processing reduces the 'glue' or 'binding' that helps to maintain a structured sequence of phonemes in short-term memory. I argue that this temporal coherence, the metaphoric glue or binding, is replaced by musical form. As we know, some songs stick in our memories.

No loss of semantic memory

Repetition ability depends in part on semantic memory remaining intact. If the conceptual contents of semantic memory are lost as a function of Alzheimer's disease, meaningfulness of stimuli should have progressively less effect on the ability to repeat as the disease worsens. Bayles, Tomoeda and Rein (1996) designed a study to evaluate the effects of meaningfulness and length of phrasal stimuli on repetition ability in mild and moderate cases of Alzheimer's disease patients and normal elderly subjects. Bayles *et al.* gave 57 Alzheimer's disease patients and 52 normal subjects six- and nine-syllable phrases that were meaningful, improbable in meaning, or meaningless. Cross-sectional and longitudinal data analyses were conducted and results failed to confirm a performance pattern consistent with a semantic memory loss theory.

Several lines of evidence suggest that in Alzheimer's disease there is a progressive degradation of the hierarchical organization of semantic memory. When clustering and switching on phonemic and semantic fluency tasks were correlated with the numbers of correct words generated on both fluency tests, the contribution of clustering was greater on the semantic task. Patients with Alzheimer's disease generated fewer correct words and made fewer switches than controls on both fluency tests. The average size of their semantic clusters was smaller and the contribution of clustering to word generation was less than for controls. Severity of dementia was correlated with the numbers of correct words and switches, but not with cluster size. The structure of semantic memory in Alzheimer's disease is probably degraded but there is no evidence that this process is progressive. Instead, progressive worsening of verbal fluency in Alzheimer's disease seems to be associated with the deterioration of mechanisms that govern initiation of search for appropriate subcategories (Beatty *et al.* 1997b). This pattern can be interpreted as reflecting significantly impaired procedural routines in Alzheimer's disease, with relative sparing of the structure of semantic memory (Chenery 1996).

No loss of source memory

A source memory task, using everyday objects in actions performed by either the participant or the experimenter, was given to probable Alzheimer's disease and elderly normal individuals. When the overall recognition performance of the two groups was made equivalent by increasing the test delay intervals for the control group, both groups of participants showed similar patterns of correct and incorrect responses. Moreover, both groups showed evidence of a generation effect and of an advantage for items repeated at study. The findings of this study suggest that, for a given level of event memory, memory for the source of the events is comparable between elderly normal and individuals with Alzheimer's disease (Brustrom and Ober 1996).

Contextual cues

Two experiments examined whether impairments in recognition memory in early stage Alzheimer's disease were due to deficits in encoding contextual information. Normal elderly people and patients diagnosed with mild stage Alzheimer's disease learned one of two tasks. In an initial experiment, correct recognition memory required participants to remember not only what items they had experienced on a given trial but also when they had experienced them. A second experiment required that participants remembered only what they had seen, not when they had seen it. Large recognition memory differences were found between the Alzheimer's disease patients and the normal elderly groups in the experiment where time tagging was crucial for successful performance. In the second experiment where the only requisite for successful recognition was remembering what one had experienced, memory of the temporal record was not necessary for successful performance. In this instance, recognition memory for the both groups was identical. Memory deficits found in early stage Alzheimer's disease may be partly due to impaired processing of contextual cues that provide crucial information about when events occur (Rickert et al. 1998).

Foster (1998) carried out a series of studies of background auditory conditions that provided such a context, and their influence upon autobiographical memory. While the use of background music has no effect on word-list recall in normal elderly people, there is a constant beneficial effect of music for autobiographical memory for patients with Alzheimer's disease. This music did not have to be familiar to the sufferer, nor did it reduce anxiety. The effect of music is stronger in cognitively impaired participants thus promoting another reason for using music-based interventions in treatment initiatives. Foster (1998), like Aldridge (1993a), argues for the use of music in assessment procedures.

As part of a programme of studies investigating memory for everyday tasks, Rusted *et al.* (1997) examined the potential of auditory and olfactory sensory cues to improve free recall of an action event (cooking an omelette) by individuals with dementia of the Alzheimer's type. Both healthy elderly people and volunteers with Alzheimer's disease recalled more of the individual actions that comprised the event when they listened, prior to recall, to a tape of sounds associated with the event. Olfactory cues which accompanied auditory cues did not produce additional benefits over auditory cues alone. The pattern of recall suggests that the auditory cues improved recall of the whole event, and were not merely increasing recall of the specific actions associated with the sound cues. Individuals with Alzheimer's disease continue to encode experiences using a combination of senses, and that they can subsequently use this sensory information to aid memory. These findings have practical implications for accessing residual memory for a wide range of therapeutic activities using the creative arts that emphasize sensory abilities.

Functional plasticity

Conscious recall of past events that have specific temporal and spatial contexts, termed episodic memory, is mediated by a system of interrelated brain regions. In Alzheimer's disease this system breaks down, resulting in an inability to recall events from the immediate past. Using brain-scanning techniques of cerebral blood flow, Becker *et al.* (1996) demonstrate that Alzheimer's disease patients show a greater activation of regions of the cerebral cortex normally involved in auditory-verbal memory, as well as activation of cortical areas not activated by normal elderly subjects. These results provide clear evidence of functional plasticity in the brain of sufferers, even if those changes do not result in normal memory function, and provide insights into the mechanisms by which the brain attempts to compensate for neurodegeneration. Similarly, it has been demonstrated that Alzheimer's disease patients can effectively learn and retain a motor skill for at least one month (Dick *et al.* 1995).

Both anterograde and retrograde procedural memory appear to be spared in Alzheimer's disease (Crystal, Grober and Masur 1989). An 82-year-old musician with Alzheimer's disease showed a preserved ability to play previously learned piano compositions from memory while being unable to identify the composer or titles of each work. He also showed a preserved ability to learn the new skill of mirror reading while being unable to recall or recognize new information.

Similar findings of creative abilities being promoted are reflected in the work of Gudrun Aldridge, Fraser Simpson and Connie Tomaino in Chapters 7, 8 and 10.

Communication

Characteristic features of communication breakdown and repair among individuals with dementia of the Alzheimer's type and their caregivers have been described by Orange *et al.* (1998). The nature of communication breakdown, how it is signalled, how it is repaired and the outcome of the repair process appear to be disease stage-dependent. Couples in the early and middle stage of the disease achieve success in resolving communication breakdowns despite declining cognitive, linguistic and conversation abilities of the individuals with the disease. This has important implications for understanding the influence of the progression of Alzheimer's disease on conversational performance and for advancing the development of communication enhancement education and training programmes for spousal caregivers of individuals with Alzheimer's disease. Music therapy will have an important role to play here as the ground of communication, as we have seen, is inherently musical. Dementia sufferers appear to be open to musical stimuli and responsive to music-making, thus implementation of musical elements in facilitating communication and expression can be enhanced as the disease progresses. If music enhances communicative abilities – indeed, is the fundamental of communication – and spousal caregivers are important in managing the progress of the disease, then we have to return to the idea that it is the caregivers who will benefit from music therapy.

Health care has an ecology. Few of us suffer alone. When we suffer, those whom we love, and love us in return, are mutually affected. Maybe we can through our endeavours restore those singing duos and bring back those dancing partners together. In a time of managed care, this will be a challenge to creative arts therapists.

CHAPTER 2

An Overview of the Music Therapy Literature Relating to Elderly People

Melissa Brotons

The number and proportion of people in the United States over the age of 65 has grown steadily during the twentieth century. Subsequently, the need to understand and address the physical, psychological and social needs of elderly people has been a topic of interest among many health-care professionals. As the prevalence of dementia increases dramatically with age, elderly people represent the largest population manifesting dementia (Aronson, Post and Guastadisegni 1993).

According to the Alzheimer's Disease and Related Disorders Association there are over 4 million Americans with dementia of the Alzheimer's type (DAT). Between the ages of 65 and 74, about 3 per cent of individuals are affected with DAT, between the ages of 75 and 84 that number increases to 19 per cent, and DAT affects over 47 per cent of individuals over the age of 85. The fact is that the American population is ageing and the fastest growing group is comprised of individuals over 85 years old (Alzheimer's Disease and Related Disorders Association 1998).

The DSM-IV (American Psychiatric Association 1994) defines the clinical syndrome of dementia as an impairment in cognitive functioning manifested in deficits in short- and long-term memory, abstract thinking, impaired judgement, language (aphasia) and personality change. The disturbance may become severe enough to interfere significantly with work or usual social activities or relationships with others. A conclusive diagnosis for

DAT does not occur until the person's brain tissue is examined after death, and at the present time there is no known cure.

Prior to the late 1980s the literature addressing clinical situations described a largely undifferentiated dementia population. However, towards the end of the decade professionals started referencing and paying more attention specifically to DAT (Prickett 1996), also known as senile dementia of the Alzheimer's type (SDAT) and Alzheimer's disease and related disorders (ADRD). There is no doubt that this population presents serious challenges in their everyday care; although there is no cure, much can be done to alleviate their problems and improve their quality of life.

Anecdotes and informal reports by health-care professionals and family members suggest that music and music therapy may have a unique effect and function on people with dementias, and more specifically on those with a probable diagnosis of ADRD (Cooper 1991; Lloyd 1992; B. Smith, 1992). These reports, presented either verbally or through association newsletters, as well as the testimonials presented at the senate hearing (Special Committee on Aging, United States Senate 1991), triggered an increasing number of research studies in the 1990s. Those studies examine the different aspects of music and the use of music therapy in the treatment of older people with ADRD in a more systematic fashion. Although references vary in the specific labelling of this population, the abbreviation ADRD will be used in the remainder of this chapter.

The purpose of this chapter is to report the results of an extensive review of literature published in the area of music and music therapy (MT) and dementias from 1980 to 1998, and to summarize the research outcomes in order to outline recommendations that may be used in clinical practice as well as in future research in this area.

While studies in the area of music/music therapy and dementias continue to accumulate, an initial study screened a total of 69 references (Brotons *et al.* 1997). Later, 12 additional references published since 1996 were reviewed and analysed resulting in a total of 81 studies.

Method

The population for this analysis of literature was defined as all published references, in refereed journals, written in English, addressing the use of music/music therapy with people with ADRD either as a basis for experimental studies or as a topic of a published report. The procedures to locate the published studies followed the steps as listed below:

1. A complete search of the Journal of Music Therapy and Music Therapy Perspectives from 1980 to the present was conducted.

2. On-line database searches including MEDLINE (1975 to present), Psychlit (1974–1998), MBI database of MuSICA (Music and Science Information Computer Archive (no information on dates covered), UNCOVER (1988 to present) and Dissertation Abstracts (1950 to present). Although the Dissertation Abstracts database was searched, master theses and dissertations located will not be included in this chapter.

A total of 81 references were identified. Of these, 50 were empirical studies, including 35 clinical empirical reports (including experimental, descriptive or case studies) using music as a therapeutic intervention (independent variable). The clinical empirical research studies were categorized according to the functional areas (dependent variable) addressed: (a) participation/preferences for music activities (n = 12), (b) social/emotional skills (n = 6), (c) cognitive skills (n = 3) and (d) behaviour management (n = 14). The remaining 12 empirical studies either were in the area of assessment or involved music cognition from a neuropsychological perspective. Narrative studies and anecdotal accounts of music therapy or articles describing non-music objectives taught through music numbered 8. Theoretical/philosophical papers describing and recommending music techniques as an alternative treatment for a variety of therapeutic objectives totalled 23. Table 2.1 gives a complete list in chronological order of the references located including author(s), year of publication, type of professionals writing the paper, type of paper, and area of functioning addressed in the paper.

Table 2.1 Complete list of references in chronological order

Authors	Year	Profession	Orientation	Content
Bright	1986	RMT	Anecdotal	Behaviour management
Geula	1986	RMT	Theoretical/philosophical	Music for self-communication
Norberg, Melin and Asplund	1986	RN	Clinical/empirical	Reactions to music
Shively and Henkin	1986	RMT	Anecdotal	Reports on the benefits of a programme that combines music dance/movement therapy
G. Smith	1986	RMT	Clinical/empirical	Cognitive skills
Beatty et al.	1988	NS	Empirical	Music cognition
Walton et al.	1988	NS	Theoretical/philosophical	Music cognition
Crystal et al.	1989	NS	Empirical	Preservation of abilities
Olderog, Millard and Smith	1989	RMT	Clinical/empirical	Social behaviour empirical
Swartz et al.	1989	NS	Empirical	Music cognition
Clair and Bernstein	1990a	RMT	Clinical/empirical	Participation in music activities
Clair and Bernstein	1990b	RMT	Clinical/empirical	Participation in music activities

Table 2.1 Complete list of references in chronological order (continued…)

Authors	Year	Profession	Orientation	Content
McCloskey	1990	Musician/consultant	Theoretical/philosophical	Report on the power of music reminiscence and life review
S. Smith	1990	RMT-BC	Theoretical/philosophical	Report on the unique power of music
Clair	1991	RMT	Anecdotal	Response to music therapy
Clayton	1991	Chaplain	Theoretical/philosophical	Describes a new approach to worship
Cooper	1991	Motivation therapist	Anecdotal	Report on the observed benefits of music
Gaebler and Hemsley	1991	NS	Clinical/empirical	Participation/mood change empirical
Prickett and Moore	1991	RMT	Clinical/empirical	Cognitive
Sacks and Tomaino	1991	MD & CMT	Theoretical/philosophical	Benefits of MT on neurological impairment
Aldridge and Aldridge	1992	Psych	Theoretical/philosophical	Position paper, treatment rationale
Braben	1992	Student nurse	Anecdotal	Report on the benefits of music for one patient
Christie	1992	RMT	Clinical/empirical	Attending skills/participation

Table 2.1 Complete list of references in chronological order (continued…)

Authors	Year	Profession	Orientation	Content
Glynn	1992	RN	Clinical/empirical	Evaluation/assessment of MT intervention
Johnson et al.	1992	CATs	Theoretical/philosophical	Position paper on the benefits of creative arts
Lindenmuth, Patel and Chang	1992	NS	Clinical/empirical	Behaviour management
Lipe	1992	RMT-BC	Theoretical/philosophical	Debate on a previously published article
Lloyd	1992	RGN	Anecdotal	Report on the benefits of music on one patient
Pollack and Namazi	1992	RMT	Clinical/empirical	Social behaviour
B. Smith	1992	SW	Anecdotal	Anecdotes on the benefits of arts programmes for ADRD
Swartz et al.	1992	NS	Theoretical/philosophical	Report on ERP measure to study brain activity
Aldridge	1993a	Psych	Theoretical/philosophical	Position paper/summary on the benefits of music therapy for assessment and treatment

Table 2.1 Complete list of references in chronological order (continued...)

Authors	Year	Profession	Orientation	Content
Clair and Bernstein	1993	RMT	Clinical/empirical	Preference for music activity
Clair, Tebb and Bernstein	1993	RMT	Clinical/empirical	Caregivers' loneliness and self-esteem, social skills
Fitzgerald-Cloutier	1993	RMT	Clinical/empirical	Behaviour management
Gerdner and Swanson	1993	RN	Clinical/empirical	Behaviour management
Groene	1993	RMT	Clinical/empirical	Behaviour management
Gunther et al.	1993	MD	Empirical	Brain mapping
Lord and Garner	1993	NS	Clinical/empirical	Social skills and cognitive (recall of past life experiences)
McLean	1993	RMT-BC	Theoretical/philosophical	Debate on a previously published article
Newman and Ward	1993	RN	Clinical/empirical	Social behaviour/positive behaviours
Polk and Kerstesz	1993	NS	Clinical/empirical	Music cognition
Pomeroy	1993	PT	Empirical	Physiotherapy

Table 2.1 Complete list of references in chronological order (continued...)

Authors	Year	Profession	Orientation	Content
Aldridge	1994	Psych	Theoretical/philosophical	Music for assessment and treatment
Beatty et al.	1994	Psych	Anecdotal	Music cognition
Bonder	1994	NS	Theoretical/philosophical	Treatment rationale
Brotons and Pickett-Cooper	1994	RMT	Clinical/empirical	Participation, preference for music activities
Casby and Holm	1994	OTR/L	Clinical/empirical	Behaviour management
Clair and Bernstein	1994	RMT	Clinical/empirical	Behaviour management
Goddaer and Abraham	1994	RN	Clinical/empirical	Behaviour management
Pomeroy	1994	PT	Empirical	Physiotherapy
Smith-Marchese	1994	Psych	Clinical/empirical	Social/emotional skills
Tappen	1994	RN	Empirical	Functional abilities
Whitcomb	1994	CMT	Theoretical	Suggestions for MT strategies
York	1994	NS	Empirical	MT assessment

Table 2.1 Complete list of references in chronological order (continued…)

Authors	Year	Profession	Orientation	Content
Aldridge	1995	Psych	Theoretical/Philosophical	Treatment rationale
Bartlett, Halpern and Dowling	1995	NS	Empirical	Music cognition
Christie	1995	RMT	Clinical/empirical	Group participation
Clair, Bernstein and Johnson	1995	RMT	Clinical/empirical	Rhythm participation characteristics
Hanser and Clair	1995	RMT	Theoretical/philosophical	Participation socialization and caregivers
Lipe	1995	RMT	Empirical	Cognitive music functioning
Sambandham and Schirm	1995	RN	Clinical/empirical	Social skills and cognitive
Silber and Hes	1995	RMT	Theoretical/philosophical	Description of song writing experience
Tabloski, McKinnon-Howe and Remington	1995	RN	Clinical/empirical	Behaviour management
Brotons and Pickett-Cooper	1996	RMT	Clinical/empirical	Behaviour management
Clair	1996b	RMT	Clinical/empirical	Participation/preferences for music activities

Table 2.1 Complete list of references in chronological order (continued…)

Authors	Year	Profession	Orientation	Content
Hanson et al.	1996	RMT	Clinical/empirical	Quality of participation
Ragneskog et al.	1996a	RN	Clinical/empirical	Behaviour management
Ragneskog et al.	1996b	RN	Clinical/empirical	Behaviour management
Beatty et al.	1997a	Psych	Anecdotal	Music cognition
Brotons et al.	1997	RMT	Literature review	Music/MT with dementias
Carruth	1997	RMT	Clinical/empirical	Cognitive
Clair and Ebberts	1997	RMT	Clinical/empirical	Participation/social/emotional
Denney	1997	RN	Clinical/empirical	Behaviour management
Kneafsey	1997	Student nurse	Literature review	Therapeutic uses of music
Korb	1997	RMT	Clinical/empirical	Participation/social skills
Thomas, Heitman and Alexander	1997	RT	Clinical/empirical	Behaviour management
Aldridge	1998b	Psych	Theoretical/philosophical	Position paper/treatment rationale
Groene et al.	1998	RMT	Clinical/empirical	Participation

Notes:

BC: board certified; CATs: creative arts therapists; CMT: certified music therapist; ERPs: event-related potentials; MD: medical doctor; NS: not specified; OTR/L: occupational therapist; Psych: psychologist; PT: physical therapist; RMT: professional music therapist; RN/RGN: registered nurse/registered general nurse; RT: recreational therapist; SW: social worker.

Literature review and analysis

General responses of dementia patients to music

The responsiveness of patients with dementia, and specifically of those with Alzheimer's disease, to music is well documented in the literature (Aldridge 1992; Kneafsey 1997). There are multiple references that report the fact that people with ADRD, despite aphasia and memory loss, continue to sing old songs (Braben 1992) and to dance to old tunes, suggesting that music may be a communication channel for reminiscing and life review (Geula 1986; McCloskey 1990). Another interesting finding is that while language deteriorates, musical abilities appear to be preserved (Swartz *et al.* 1989). Case studies included those involving individuals who retain the ability to play previously learned compositions but who are unable to identify the composer or titles of the work (Crystal *et al.* 1989) or unable to name previously heard songs when they are played back (Beatty *et al.* 1988; Beatty *et al.* 1994; Beatty L, Brumback and Vonsattel 1997). Further, a variety of preserved cognitive skills were reported in five patients with dementia, including a maintained ability to play trombone in a Dixieland band. Beatty *et al.* (1988) interpreted these findings as deficits in anterograde recall and recognition and in remote memory in the patients, while retention of motor skills was considered intact. These findings are consistent with the dissociation between declarative and procedural memory observed in amnesics (Cohen and Squire 1980) as they illustrate a very well preserved procedural (or motor skill) memory for musical performance among musicians with a diagnosis of ADRD. However, it appears that their declarative semantic memory for music, and language associated with it, is severely impaired in these ADRD patients.

Bartlett *et al.* (1995) conducted a series of experiments to compare the performance of ADRD, normal elderly people and younger adults in recognizing familiar and unfamiliar melodies in order to understand better the declarative memory deficits that elderly patients with ADRD seem to present. Results demonstrated that ADRD patients are more impaired relative to controls in recognition memory for well-known tunes, and that deficits in recognition memory are not necessarily continuous across age and severity of ADRD.

The functional dissociation of declarative and procedural memory implies differential underlying neural substrates, with ADRD affecting some brain systems more than others; a premise that has received much empirical support (many reviews exist on this topic; for a fairly comprehensive and current treatise, see Khachaturian and Radebaugh 1996). Although most descriptions of the declarative/procedural dichotomy are hierarchical, with declarative knowledge viewed as more complex or recent evolutionarily (Squire 1987), a dissociation between language and musical abilities in ADRD may reflect differential hemispheric degeneration. For example, Polk and Kerstesz (1993) administered a series of standardized language batteries and music tasks to two musicians with possible ADRD and lateralized cortical atrophy. Subject 1, who presented greater left cortical atrophy and primary progressive aphasia (including non-fluent and content-impaired speech), showed fluent musical production including melodic and rhythmic structures. Conversely, Subject 2 manifested greater right hemisphere involvement and spared language abilities, while this subject's musical performance was deficient in melodic and rhythmic production. These results support a dissociation between left and right hemispheric contributions to language and music functions, respectively.

Other recent neuropsychological investigations of ADRD patients have utilized topographic brain-mapping techniques, which enable the assessment of neural activity while an individual is involved in a cognitive task such as music perception. Such bio-behavioural analyses of responsiveness to music involve correlating physiological measures such as electroencephalographs (EEGs) and cognitive or motor task performance (Gunther et al. 1993) and have enhanced the value of EEG in clinical diagnosis (Walton et al. 1988). For example, Swartz et al. (1992) compared Potential 3 event-related potentials (ERP) and performance on music perception tasks between older healthy subjects and those with ADRD. Results indicated that subjects with ADRD showed slower P3 latencies and were less accurate overall on the task than were the healthy subjects. The authors concluded, however, that if the putative role of the P3 ERP is valid, the existence of this physiological response in ADRD patients suggests that they may maintain the ability to attend to and discriminate differences in fundamental music elements such as pure tones, timbre, and interval series (melodic elements).

As a whole, this research suggests that music processing which is preserved in ADRD may be occurring in different parts of the brain than familiar linguistic mechanisms. Further, these regions may be the last to deteriorate in the disease process, at least in a subset of ADRD patients. Because the creative arts therapies in general, and music therapy specifically, rely less on verbal processing, they may offer a unique approach to accessing stored knowledge and memories that control certain behaviours.

Treatment programmes

Numerous informal observations led to the belief that music may offer a unique component to the treatment of elderly patients with ADRD (Aldridge 1993a; Christie 1992). Music therapy interventions have been used with dementia patients within a cognitive-behavioural as well as psycho-therapeutic context for the purpose of improving and maintaining cognitive, physical and emotional skills such as reorientation, exercise/physiotherapy, maintenance of social behaviours, receptive and expressive language skills, anxiety reduction, maintenance of memory functions, increased positive affect and creative self-expression. Music apparently has the power to provide the Alzheimer's patient with a sense of accomplishment, to energize and stimulate, to trigger words, and to soothe and comfort both the patient and caregiver (Pomeroy 1993, 1994; S. Smith 1990; Tappen 1994). Further, music may ameliorate some of the behavioural and emotional consequences of ADRD, especially as a later-stage intervention (Bonder 1994; Bright 1986). Sacks and Tomaino (1991) postulate that music for patients with dementia acts as a 'sort of Proustian mnemonic, eliciting emotions and associations that had been forgotten, giving the patient access once again to moods and memories, thoughts and worlds that seemingly had been forgotten' (p. 11). They emphasize the importance of selecting music that will have significance and meaning for each individual in order to produce an effect.

Several references in the literature include specific programme descriptions listing all the benefits for those with ADRD as witnessed by the authors. Shively and Henkin (1986) describe a programme that combines music and movement therapy with ADRD clients. By centring around a specific topic, they report the benefits of this type of programme such as to

> provide reality orientation; a non-threatening environment for those who feel unsecure and unsafe; a means for creative expression for those who find it difficult to communicate; a therapeutic environment for those who become agitated or need structure; and stimulation to help maintain mental and physical capabilities for the forgetful and less mobile person. (Shively and Henkin 1986, p.56)

Whitcomb (1994) recommends the use of a variety of music activities as well as therapeutic strategies with ADRD patients in order to reduce tension, restlessness, agitation, depression, confusion, fear, feelings of loneliness, isolation and low self-esteem. Similarly, Johnson *et al.* (1992) describe group work involving the creative arts therapies on an Alzheimer's unit. They believe that the non-verbal essence of art, dance and music therapy, and their focus on sensory and affective experiences, make them effective approaches to encourage reminiscence, self-expression and socialization. Clayton (1991) describes a new approach to worship for Alzheimer's patients and their families in which music is one of the stressed elements to make the experience more meaningful.

Clinical empirical studies

The previous section includes a wealth of programme proposals and accounts of the potential benefits of music in general and of music therapy in particular to address a variety of issues with patients with ADRD. This leads to the question, 'Is there empirical evidence of the effectiveness of this approach?' The following sections will review empirical studies utilising music therapy interventions with ADRD subjects. Tables 2.2, 2.3, 2.4 and 2.5 will identify specific objectives addressed by each study.

Assessment / evaluation

Dementia and its progression has been assessed and diagnosed through a brief cognitive test, the Mini-Mental State Examination (MMSE), which evaluates various functional capabilities and is based on questions and activities (Folstein, Folstein and McHugh 1975). Although this test is widely used, it has been criticized because of its failure to discriminate minor language deficits and neglects to assess fluency and intentionality (Aldridge and Aldridge 1992). The use of music therapy, specifically a dynamic musical play such as improvisation, may be utilized to stimulate cognitive function and elicit some of the language responses that the MMSE fails to evaluate including the fluency of musical production and those prosodic elements of speech production which are not lexically dependent (Aldridge and Aldridge 1992). Further, improvised music enables an evaluation of intentionality, attention, concentration and perseverance on the task at hand, as well as episodic memory of ADRD patients (A. Aldridge 1995; D. Aldridge 1994, 1998b; D. Aldridge and G. Aldridge 1992).

Although there are, at the present time, no standardized measures for evaluating the specific effects of music therapy on patients with a diagnosis of ADRD, there are several studies that are aimed at testing the psychometric properties of newly developed music therapy assessment tools. Bruscia (1995) defines

> assessment studies as those aimed at gaining insights about individual clients or client population served by music therapy – their conditions, problems, resources, experiences, and therapeutic needs...a music therapy assessment study reveals how clients listen to, make, experience, or otherwise respond to music under various conditions, and relates these data to their conditions, problems, resources, experiences, and therapeutic needs. (Bruscia 1995, p.18)

York (1994) developed a quantitative music therapy test, the Residual Music Skills Test (RMST) to measure musical capabilities of persons with probable Alzheimer's disease. The objective of this test is to measure music skills that people would normally obtain over a lifetime without having been exposed to formal music education. The musical subsections of the test included the following: (a) recall of song task, (b) instrument identification task, (c) tonal memory task, (d) recall of instrument name, and (e) musical language. The preliminary field testing results of this tool, which included correlations with the MMSE, suggest that the RMST may be measuring unique cognitive functions such as actual music processing in the brain. In another study, Lipe (1995) developed and evaluated a measure focusing on the performance of musical tasks for evaluation of cognitive functioning, and assessing the relationship between music background and music task performance of older adults with ADRD. Subjects' data were collected through MMSE, the Brief Cognitive Rating Scale (BCRS), the Severe Impairment Battery (SIB), and 19 specially designed music performance tasks which included verbal, singing and rhythm skills. Results showed that music background was not related to music task performance. Conversely, there appears to be a strong indication that those individuals without dementia scored higher in the music performance tasks than those with a diagnosis of dementia.

Glynn (1992) developed a music therapy assessment tool (MTAT) to evaluate the effects of music therapy on behavioural patterns (physical, psychological and social) of ADRD patients. It includes three sections, with Part I designed to be administered during the music intervention, and Parts II and III after the music intervention. To test the MTAT for internal consistency and inter-rater reliability, 20 subjects identified as having severe cognitive decline were exposed to 30 minutes of selected taped music. Although the results revealed a high inter-rater reliability and internal consistency reliability, several notes have appeared in refereed journals questioning the methodology and validity of this study (Lipe 1992; McLean 1993). This reaction may be due to a statement in the discussion section of Glynn's paper in which the author postulates that 'nurses need not be musicians to achieve a positive effect. Music can be presented by means of a tape, compact disc, or a record or it can be played or sung live' (p.9), thus reducing music to playing taped music while ignoring the importance of professional training to design and implement music therapy interventions.

Participation/preferences for music activities

The importance of choosing and adapting music activities to maximize participation, and consequently to achieve therapeutic objectives, is stressed by professional music therapists. In addition, the significance of assessing patients' music preferences as a basis to choose music for the interventions has also been noted (Moore, Staum and Brotons 1992). Several empirical studies in the area of music/music therapy and dementias have addressed these issues. Norberg *et al.* (1986) observed reactions (i.e. mouth movement, eye opening, eye blinking, verbal reactions, pulse and respiration rates, and hand and foot movements) of two patients in the final stages of DAT when stimulated with music, touch and object presentation. The subjects' reactions to music differed from those to touch, and object presentation with one of the subjects appearing to show more of an orientation response and the other more relaxation to music; the authors admit, however, the subjectivity of these observations. Gaebler and Hemsley (1991) also used music stimulation on six patients with severe dementia to observe its effect on behavioural and emotional responses. Although their findings showed considerable variability among subjects, there were clear effects on four out of six patients. Clair (1996b) compared the effect of singing, reading and silence on alert responses of late stage dementia patients. She provided four individual sessions, in sequential days, and observed that more alert responses were exhibited during singing than reading or silence, although this difference did not reach statistical significance. Another important finding in this study was that responses tended to increase over time, indicating that time may be an important factor for evoking responses from this population.

A number of other studies have investigated preference and participation in a variety of music activities (Brotons and Pickett-Copper 1994; Christie 1992; Clair and Bernstein 1990a, 1990b). Participation appeared to be significantly longer for instrument playing, dance/movement activities and playing games than for composition/improvisation (Brotons and

Pickett-Copper 1994). Comparably, Clair and Bernstein (1990b) found that subjects participated longer during instrument playing work (particularly vibrotactile playing) than during singing, indicating that singing may tend to decrease as the dementia progresses. No differences were observed for preferences between vibrotactile and auditory stimuli, nor did stimulus preference interact with type of dementia (ADRD or dementia due to alcohol abuse) in a later study (Clair and Bernstein 1993); however, these subjects lay on the bed for the entire duration of the sessions when their usual behaviour was to wander and move around.

Another study reported that purposeful responses occurred significantly more during movement than during singing activities for three different stages of cognitive functioning, as assessed by the Global Deterioration Scale (GDS: Hanson et al. 1996). When rhythm and singing activities were presented at low level demand, participants appeared significantly more involved. Although no differences were observed for level of cognitive functioning across activity type, patients manifesting greatest cognitive decline (GDS 5–6) spent proportionately more time engaged in passive disruption than subjects at higher cognitive levels, particularly during rhythm and singing activities. Similar results were reported by Groene et al. (1998) in a study conducted with a group of ADRD patients in stages 5 and 6 of the GDS. This group had a significantly higher incidence of purposeful responses during exercise sessions than during sing-along sessions. Another important finding in this study was the effect of time spent by the therapist playing the guitar and singing on the duration of patients' participation.

Clair et al. (1995) described rhythm-playing characteristics in ADRD, specifically as it refers to type of drum preferred, entrainment of playing, imitation of drum strokes, and complexity of rhythm patterns produced. They found that the subjects increased significantly in their imitation of progressively more complex rhythm patterns. Furthermore, it appeared that participation was higher with the floor tom followed by bass, paddle and frame drums, respectively. Entrainment playing increased significantly from baseline to Experimental Session 1, then it was maintained across the experimental sessions and dropped dramatically from the last experimental to the return to baseline sessions; thus, performance of this activity seemed to be dependent on the presence of the therapist rather than reflecting a learned response.

Although it is not empirically based, Silber and Hes (1995) described the successful experience of using songwriting with patients diagnosed with

Table 2.2 Clinical/empirical research on music with Alzheimer's disease and related disorders: participation/preference for music activities

Authors	Year	Target behaviour(s)
Norberg *et al.*	1986	Eye blinking Eye open Verbal reactions Mouth movement Heart and respiration rates Hand and foot movement
Clair and Bernstein	1990a	Purposeful participation Consistency of participation
Clair and Bernstein	1990b	Duration of participation
Gaebler and Hemsley	1991	Engagement Emotional response
Christie	1992	Duration of participation
Clair and Bernstein	1993	Preference: duration of choice
Brotons and Pickett-Cooper	1994	Time participating Verbal report
Clair *et al.*	1995	Duration of participation Number of correct hand stroke imitations Frequency of entrainment playing Number and complexity of imitated rhythm
Christie	1995	Duration of participation
Hanson *et al.*	1996	Length of purposeful participation
Clair and Ebberts	1997	Frequency of participation Frequency of initiation of contact Frequency of physical responses to contact
Groene *et al.*	1998	Duration of singing/humming to songs Duration of movement/exercise

ADRD in a day-care centre in Israel. The authors state that songwriting is an activity that allows patients with ADRD to overcome partially and temporarily their cognitive, memory and language deficiencies when the activity is properly guided and adapted for the population in question by a music therapist.

The important implication is that the same music activity may not be equally suitable for all participants, as activities differ in the extent to which they require verbal, cognitive and physical skills (see Table 2.2). Although the overall results of these studies suggest that people with ADRD enjoy music activities and are capable of participating in a variety of activities, consideration of the individual's abilities is crucial for optimizing purposeful participation and reducing disruption and agitation. In addition, it is suggested that the presence of a highly participatory client in a group may be an important element to increase group participation (Christie 1995).

Social/emotional skills

Individuals with ADRD inevitably decline in cognitive and social functioning and subsequently are able to participate in fewer purposeful activities as the disorder progresses. Consequently, it seems imperative to examine the extent to which structured music activities can aid in the maintenance and even reattainment of social skills that were once part of those people's repertoire. Application of such activities will potentially delay social withdrawal, enabling patients to continue being part of their social milieu for as long as possible.

In that regard, many studies have delineated beneficial outcomes in terms of social and emotional behaviours in ADRD patients following music/ music therapy interventions. When compared to results obtained after group discussion, benefits of participation in group singing include higher vocal/ verbal participation, sitting, and walking with others during and after the intervention (Olderog-Millard and Smith 1989). Additional effects include a significant (24 per cent) increase in social behaviour (talking, vocalizing, gesturing, smiling, touching, humming, singing and whistling) from before to after individual music therapy sessions (Pollack and Namazi 1992), significantly higher scores from pre- to post-test in mood, social interaction and recall in patients who listened to music relative to those who completed puzzles or served as a control group (Lord and Garner 1993), and significant scores in solicited and unsolicited feedback and affective responses (smiling) during rhythm and singing sessions in comparison to discussion sessions

(Korb 1997). Although participation in live music also enhanced reality orientation, Smith-Marchese (1994) reported only a non-significant trend toward improved sociability in her study of ADRD patients.

Sambandham and Schirm (1995) examined the effects of participation in music activities on communication and socialization skills and the capacity to reminisce and recall memories. They found that subjects tended to talk less during music than before and after music observation periods; however, patients interacted significantly more with each other after music sessions. Furthermore, memory skills improved significantly after music sessions in those subjects with the lowest cognitive functioning levels. The authors suggested that music may be one form of communication that is preserved in persons with ADRD. This conclusion is further supported by the report of a severely regressed man diagnosed with probable ADRD who received music therapy (including singing and instrument playing) (Clair 1991). Although his physical and cognitive state deteriorated over the 15-month treatment programme, he was able to continue communicating, watching others in the group, singing at some level, interacting with instruments, and remaining seated for the duration of the music therapy sessions without much change. The author indicates that music therapy provided stimulation and an opportunity to come out of his isolation, at least for short periods of time.

Home care seems to be the choice for the majority of people with dementias (Gilhooly and Birren 1986). Subsequently, caregivers suddenly face a whole set of problems and demands which often require new adjustments and routines, a transition which may be facilitated by music therapy. Although Clair et al. (1993) did not observe significant differences in caregivers' loneliness and self-esteem scores from the beginning to the end of a music therapy intervention, caregivers reported that it was an opportunity for them to learn about new resources that could be used to enhance their relationship with their spouses. In a later publication, Hanser and Clair (1995) describe in great detail two programmes for Alzheimer's patients and their caregivers with the purpose of assisting in retrieving losses and making contact among patients in the early stages of the disease and their family members, and to maintain the participation and active involvement in purposeful activities for those in the late stages of the disease. These programmes included a variety of music activities: relaxation exercises to music, singing, instrument playing, improvisation and songwriting. Although no empirical information is included in this report, both programmes were qualified as successful by staff and family members. Clair and Ebberts (1997) studied the effect of singing, dancing and rhythm playing on the participation and social behaviours (i.e. initiating touch and responding to touch) of patients in late stage dementia and their caregivers. Both patients and caregivers participated the most during rhythm-playing activities. Caregivers initiated touch more frequently than the patients but the patients showed a greater response to touch. Furthermore, although results did not show significant differences between pre-test and post-test scores in the caregivers' burden, positive/negative affect, depression and self-reported health, except for satisfaction with visits, their satisfaction with visits in music therapy reached significance, as compared to visits before music therapy.

Another study (Newman and Ward 1993) observed the effect on social/positive behaviours of ADRD patients participating in intergenerational music activities. That is, subjects were observed while participating in music activities with and without the presence of a group of pre-schoolers. Behaviours observed included smiling, extending hands, clapping hands, tapping feet, singing, interacting verbally, touching, hugging and holding hands. There was a significant increase in two spontaneous behaviours, touching and extending hands, when the children were present, and a

Table 2.3 Clinical/empirical research on music with Alzheimer's disease and related disorders: social skills

Authors	Year	Target behaviour(s)
Olderog-Millard and Smith	1989	Frequency of social behaviour
Pollack and Namazi	1992	Frequency of social behaviour
Clair et al.	1993	UCLA loneliness scales scores Rasenberg self-esteem scores
Lord and Garner	1993	Recall Interaction Mood
Newman and Ward	1993	Positive behaviours: smiling, touching, eye-contact, hugging, extending hands
Sambandhan and Schirm	1995	Communication Socialization Recall

significant increase in holding hands (a direction given by the music therapist) when children were not present.

It is important to remember how difficult it is to elicit any behaviour from people with dementia, much less to observe spontaneous positive interactions with other people. These studies illustrate that social behaviours can occur among clients with ADRD when the setting and environment is properly structured, and that music therapy interventions can foster and enhance these types of behaviours (see Table 2.3).

Cognitive skills

Decline of cognitive functioning is one of the most salient and earliest features of ADRD. Amnesia, aphasia, apraxia, agnosia and anomia are a few of the more common cognitive symptoms seen in patients with ADRD (Scruggs 1991). As cognitive skills are progressively lost, agitation and severe behaviour problems are usually manifested. At the present time ADRD is an irreversible disease with no cure, but neurological studies mentioned in a previous section of this chapter suggest that cognitive processes related to music processing may be preserved, even in the latest stages of the disease. Therefore, music may function as a catalyst to exercise and maintain other parallel non-musical processes (Aldridge 1998b). Unfortunately, very few references specifically address the effects of music on cognitive processes. Several of the studies, however, examined overall cognitive functioning in addition to other abilities. It is interesting to note, though, that the few reports identified suggest that music may enhance language and memory skills. (Note that some of the studies were described in the previous section, with recall and cognitive functioning as dependent variables.)

Prickett and Moore (1991) found that patients remembered the words of songs they had sung during therapy sessions better than spoken material, and that the percentage of recall was better for older than for newer songs. This study also seems to suggest that, with enough repetition, subjects were capable of learning new material when presented in the context of a song. Another study compared three treatment interventions: musically cued reminiscence, verbally cued reminiscence, and music activity participation cognitive functioning as measured by the MMSE (G. Smith 1986). Overall MMSE scores improved following music activities sessions, but not the other two interventions. Scores on the language subscales of the MMSE improved following the musically and verbally cued reminiscence treatments.

In a later study, Carruth (1997) reported the improvement in the naming abilities (face–name recognition) of ADRD patients when tested with the spaced-retrieval technique that participated in individual singing and conversation sessions. For four of the seven participants in the study, singing improved the percentage of correct recognition responses in comparison to the non-music condition. Perhaps the most revealing finding in this study was that five of the seven subjects were able to recall the name of the targeted person after more than one day from the music condition, suggesting their ability to retain novel information for longer periods of time (see Table 2.4).

Table 2.4 Clinical/empirical research on music with Alzheimer's disease and related disorders: cognitive skills

Authors	Year	Target behaviour(s)
G. Smith	1986	Cognitive functioning
Prickett and Moore	1991	Number of words recalled
Carruth	1997	Percentage correct face–name recognition responses

Behaviour management

A variety of behavioural problems frequently accompany cognitive deterioration in ADRD such as irritability, withdrawal, depression, anxiety, fear, paranoia or suspiciousness, aggression, delusions, hallucinations, wandering, pacing, agitation and sleeping problems (Cohen et al. 1993). These symptoms impose additional challenges and demands in the care of these individuals, and frequently precipitate institutionalization for those who still live at home. Supervision needs to increase in these cases to ensure patients' safety and manageability, therefore, alleviation of these problems can improve quality of life decreasing for both patients and caregivers.

Several studies in the music therapy field have empirically evaluated the uses of music for behaviour control and management, and show promise as an alternative to chemicals and restraints. For example, a significant relationship between sleep facilitation and music was observed in patients with ADRD, but not in healthy controls; thus, music may be an alternative treatment to sedative-hypnotic drugs to alleviate sleeping problems of people with ADRD (Lindenmuth *et al.* 1992). Also, a decrease in agitation in patients' agitation during bathing, as assessed by the Cohen-Mansfield Agitation Inventory, was noted specifically in the aggressive behaviour category (Thomas *et al.* 1997). Likewise, a decrease in patients' agitation, as assessed by the same previous tool, was noted during and after music therapy intervention, although the amount of improvement varied greatly among the five individuals (Gerdner and Swanson 1993). These findings suggest that music preferences are quite individualized, and obtaining specific titles of selections may be a key variable to success with this type of intervention. This is further supported by Clair and Bernstein (1994) where no significant differences in percentage of agitation were observed among conditions (background stimulative or sedative music versus no music), although agitation appeared to be significantly lower during the noon mealtime than in morning and afternoon sessions. The authors suggest that group size, music preferences and the possibility of adapting and structuring music activities on the spot are important variables when working with this population. Conversely, in more recent studies that also targeted agitation, favourable results were reported when the same tape of New Age music during meals (Goddaer and Abraham 1994) and classical music (Tabloski *et al.* 1995) was used with all the subjects throughout the treatment periods. Similarly, Casby and Holm (1994) found that two forms of taped music (classical and preferred) appeared effective in decreasing disruptive verbalizations, although the effect of preferred music was stronger.

Similarly, other studies that compared three different types of music to decrease agitation at mealtime – soothing music, popular music of the 1920s and 1930s, and popular and rock music from the 1980s – showed more favourable results with the soothing music than with the other two styles of music (Denney 1997; Ragneskog *et al.* 1996b), although it seemed that food consumption, and specifically dessert, was greater when pop music of the 1920s and 1930s was played (Ragneskog *et al.* 1996a). It therefore seems that music therapy is effective overall in reducing agitation and disruptive behaviours, but it is important to take into account the importance of music styles, subjects' preferences and the specific behaviours that are addressed.

The use of live music as a music therapy intervention also appears to be highly effective to decrease agitation. Brotons and Pickett-Cooper (1996) found that patients were significantly less agitated (i.e. manifesting reductions in pacing, hand wringing, inability to sit or lie still, rapid speech, psychomotor activity, crying and repetitive verbalizations of distress) during or after, relative to before, music therapy, and that music background did not appear related to effectiveness of treatment. The therapeutic interventions included participation in a variety of music activities: singing, playing instruments, dancing/moving to music, composition/improvisation and games. Similar studies reported that subjects tended to remain seated longer

Table 2.5 Clinical/empirical research on music with Alzheimer's disease and related disorders: behaviour management

Authors	Year	Target behaviour(s)
Scruggs	1991	Percentage time and frequency wandering Length of stay in sessions Cognition: MMSE scores
Lindenmuth *et al.*	1992	Number of hours of productive sleep Sleep patterns
Fitzgerald-Cloutier	1993	Length of wandering
Gerdner and Swanson	1993	Agitation scores
Groene	1993	Wandering
Casby and Holm	1994	Frequency of disruptive verbalizations
Clair and Bernstein	1994	Percentage agitation
Goddaer and Abraham	1994	Agitation scores
Tabloski *et al.*	1995	Agitation scores
Brotons and Pickett-Cooper	1996	Agitation scores
Ragneskog *et al.*	1996a	Amount of food Behaviour problems: irritation, fear-panic, depressed mood
Ragneskog *et al.*	1996b	Time spent with dinner Agitation behaviours
Denney	1997	Agitation behaviours during mealtime
Thomas *et al.*	1997	Agitation behaviours during bathing

during participative music therapy sessions than during reading (Fitzgerald-Cloutier 1993; Groene 1993). Further, decreases in wandering and increases in length of stay in sessions were noted following structured music activities or music listening with contingent verbal prompt (Scruggs 1991). Although the effects of the two music treatments did not differ significantly, structured music activities were more effective in reducing wandering, and the contingent music listening with verbal prompt was more effective in increasing length of stay in the sessions. There was a non-significant trend towards improvement in cognition across testing conditions, but again, both music conditions appeared to be equally effective.

The results of all these studies show the potential of the carefully planned application of music as an alternative to medication and restraints for managing behavioural problems of patients with a diagnosis of ADRD. In addition, they support the theory that altering the environment, in this case through music, can be a viable method to decrease these symptoms (see Table 2.5).

Results

Table 2.1 showed that the publication of articles concerning music/music therapy and dementias started in 1986. From 1986 to 1991 the number of publications was low, ranging from 0 to 6 per year, but from 1992 to 1994 there was a considerable jump to 12–13 publications per year, decreasing again to 10 and 5 in 1995 and 1996 respectively, and 8 and 2 in 1997 and 1998.

Concerning the authors of the publications and publication sources, it is interesting to note that except for one master's thesis, the references included in this chapter have been published in a variety of professional, refereed journals and by a variety of health professionals besides professional music therapists (see Table 2.6). Specifically 47 per cent of the publications were authored by at least one music therapist, and 53 per cent by other health professionals.

Although this review focused on studies that specifically evaluated responses of people with ADRD to music/music therapy interventions, two of the studies retrieved and included also evaluated responses of family caregivers to music interventions, perhaps indicating an initial interest in addressing the needs of this group.

Table 2.6 Frequency of publications according to type of professional	
Type of professional	Frequency of publications
Professional music therapist	38
Not specified	12
Registered nurse/registered general nurse	14
Psychologist	8
Physical therapist	2
Musician	1
Chaplain	1
Social worker	1
Occupational therapist	1
Medical doctor	1
Motivation therapist	1
Recreation therapist	1

According to the references reviewed in a previous work (Brotons *et al.* 1997) and the new ones added in this review, there was a lot of variability in the type of music techniques used in the clinical empirical studies, but some trends emerged. In the area of participation/preferences for music activities (n = 12) the majority of studies used live/active music experiences which required that a patient or a group of patients play musical instruments, sing or move with the therapist. It is obvious that in this group of studies, music functioned as structure to promote and enhance participation and determine preferences for music activities. In the area of social/emotional skills (n = 6) also the majority of the studies involved live/active music therapy in order to set the occasion for the type of social/emotional responses that the music activities intended to promote.

The three studies that specifically targeted cognitive skills used live/ active music, specifically singing. In this area, music appears to serve as an auditory cue to enhance memory and language skills. Due to the many similarities between singing and verbal language, and because of the strength of music in aiding retention and recall of information, singing seems to be the most appropriate activity for accessing these cognitive skills.

Ten of the fourteen behavioural management studies used listening to taped music as the main intervention, and the other four used structured live music activities. It therefore appears that there is a tendency to use a more passive approach for treating behaviour problems; that is, music activities are structured so that patients basically listen to live or recorded music played by the therapist. It is interesting to note that the majority of studies in this area were not conducted by professional music therapists, suggesting that there may be some relationship between type of music intervention used and type of professional implementing it.

Conclusion

A comprehensive review of literature in music and dementias revealed that clinical research in this area started basically in 1986, with the highest number of publications on this topic occurring between 1992 and 1994. An explanation for this eruption of publication may be the 1991 Senate hearing (Special Committee on Aging, United States Senate 1991) in which special funds were allocated to finance research and demonstration projects in music therapy with elderly people. Although a good portion of the literature reviewed in this chapter was authored by and involved professional music therapists, over half of the references (n = 45) were written by health professionals other than professional music therapists. Nurses, in particular, seem to be interested in the applications and potential effects of music on people with dementias. This may be a reason why the clinical empirical studies were so varied in methodology and implementation of music therapy procedures. One of the few consistencies across studies was the music selections used, when these were specified. The music repertoire selected in the studies seem to take into consideration older people's preferences, as reported in previous studies (Moore *et al.* 1992). While the profession may benefit in its development and reputation if health professionals, other than music therapists, witness and report the positive effects of music on people with dementias, it is also distressing that people without music therapy training implement music therapy programmes and convincingly write statements such as 'sophisticated skills may not be essential to achieving some success with music' (Sambandham and Schirm 1995, p.82). Certainly this is material for debate among professional music therapists (McLean 1993). A question this position introduces is: What should the role and future of professional music therapists be in caring for people with dementias, and how can it enhance nursing interventions?

Professional music therapists are accountable for providing efficient, beneficial treatment. As the Music Therapy Standards of Practice specify, the music therapist is responsible for (1) assessing, (2) designing and implementing music therapy treatments, (3) monitoring client progress, and (4) reformulating their practice according to data collected and the new advancements in the field. As Prickett (1996) states:

> It follows that clinical music therapists always face a dilemma when formulating treatment plans. On the one hand, if they wait until sufficient valid, empirical data on all aspects of a disability or music response are available before attempting to design a therapy session, they may well reach retirement age before even one client can be served. On the other hand, promulgating the efficacy of music therapy in general, or of specific music therapy techniques, in the absence of any substantiation other than intuition or tradition borders on professional recklessness. (Prickett 1996, p.145)

Review of the 38 clinical empirical studies conducted from 1986 to 1998 provide sufficient evidence to conclude that music can be structured effectively to enhance participation and social/emotional skills, and to decrease behaviour problems, as well as for use as a stimulus/prompt to aid in recall and language skills with people with ADRD. The summary of the findings is as follows:

1. Older people with a diagnosis of ADRD continue participating in structured music activities into the late stages of the disease.

2. Instrument playing and dance/movement seem to be the most preferred live music activities of people with ADRD, as these are the activities they can participate in the most and the longest, even into late stages of the disease. Although singing is a very popular and widely used activity with the geriatric population, it appears to decline over time in people with dementias. Nevertheless, they can participate in a variety of music activities when appropriately adapted to their level of functioning, even those that demand more

creativity and spontaneity such as composition/improvisation, games and songwriting.

3. Modelling of the expected responses, either by a higher function-ing peer or by the music therapist, seems to be an important element to ensure and maintain participation.

4. Individual and small group (three to five people) sessions appear to be the most successful settings for music therapy with ADRD patients.

5. Social/emotional skills, including interaction and communication can be enhanced and even improved through live structured music activities. Music therapy interventions can promote interactions and can teach ADRD patients and their caregivers new interaction skills. The presence of youngsters in music therapy sessions can be a positive addition to foster socialization and communication skills in ADRD.

6. Music can enhance cognitive skills such as memory. Information presented in a song context enhances retention and recall of information.

7. Music interventions have shown to be an effective alternative to medication and physical restraints to manage behaviour problems of ADRD. The findings of this review of literature suggest that music preference is a key element to ensure success in the music interventions.

Taken together, these findings show that people with ADRD respond to music, suggesting that music may be one medium through which elderly people with ADRD may communicate and access memories that are difficult to recall through traditional verbal means. The reason why this response occurs is not yet clear. Is it because of the aesthetic nature of music that in turn activates preserved brain structures, thereby allowing these people to connect with the outside world for certain periods of time? Or is the interpersonal, caring relationship established with a therapist responsible for eliciting the responses? Certainly, further research is warranted.

Acknowledgement

Portions of this chapter have appeared previously and are included here by permission (Brotons et al. 1997).

CHAPTER 3

Working with Words
People with Dementia
and the Significance of Narratives

Trisha Kotai-Ewers

A Great Story

We ought to write a story on this
You could go on and on for years
We'll make up a story
The whole set
You're going to have a great story
What a pity I didn't write it up all over
What is the hard part if you don't remember them
What is the pity of it if you don't remember them
It's a strange world isn't it?

Irene

Irene and I were going to 'make up a story'. That is, Irene was telling me the story. I was merely her scribe. As she said the words, I wrote them down. If I missed any I could rarely ask her to repeat herself. Irene had dementia. She could not remember the words she had just spoken. But they were her words, telling her story. And, like all our stories, hers was coloured by her personality, her emotions and especially by her passage through a disease which was slowly attacking her thought processes and memory banks. Then in her mid-eighties, Irene had lived in a dementia-specific hostel for the last six years. The phrases which make up *A Great Story* were scattered through the first conversation we had in March 1997. I had explained to her that I was working in the hostel as a writer in residence. If she gave permission I would write down her words as we spoke, and then structure them into poems. Since then she has been happy for me to record her words. A very special relationship has developed between us over time. When I visited her recently after some months' absence, there was at first no recognition. Then I turned on her the smile she once called 'That grin!' Immediately she exclaimed: 'Oh, there you are!'

Irene's response to me after such a long absence reassured me in my conclusion regarding the place of this chapter in a book on music therapy in dementia care. Planning the chapter I was confronted by a problem. How to justify writing a study of the words of people with dementia in a book devoted to music? Certainly both words and music are integral elements in the domain of song where the rhythm of words combines with the rhythm of music. It seems, however, that a more potent connection lies in the role of emotion in both art forms. The composer expresses his or her emotions through music. We, the listeners, experience an emotional response to that music. I present the words I collect in poetic form. And poetry is most often the distillation of the poet's emotional reaction into words.

Concern with the emotions of people with dementia is essentially a recent phenomenon. In the UK, its roots lie in the work of psychologist Tom Kitwood and the Bradford Dementia Research Group. The concept of personhood formulated by Kitwood (1997) extends a far wider net than the left-brain-biased definitions favoured by some moral philosophers, who see personhood residing in characteristics such as rationality, self-control and self-awareness (Post 1995, p.15). But, who could doubt the distinctive 'person-ness' of a lanky, bouncy woman who flopped into a chair exclaiming: 'I've worn the bottom off me!' Irene and the occupational therapist had been 'batting' a balloon back and forth across the hostel lounge, amid great hilarity. Now she was exhausted. These were the first of her words that I recorded in conversations at intervals over 30 months. They epitomize the idiosyncratic turn of phrase that characterizes all of her language.

Until this person-centred approach began to find a wider acceptance, discourse in dementia was largely seen as an area for diagnostic study. Once we consider people with dementia in a holistic way it becomes possible, indeed desirable, to hear what they can tell us about what is happening to them. While he does not report these actual voices, research fellow Malcolm Goldsmith in his book *Hearing the Voice of People with Dementia* (1996) quotes doctors, staff nurses and family carers with guidance on the value of hearing, and ways of listening to this voice. Meanwhile writer John Killick (1994) has been listening to and recording the words of people with dementia since December 1992. Like Goldsmith, Killick is attached to the Dementia Services Development Centre at Stirling University. My work in Western Australia has its impetus as an extension of Killick's work. At the same time approaches such as validation, reminiscence therapy and autobiographical work emphasize the importance of the spoken word while, on another level, personal stories like those of Robert Davis (1989), Diana Friel McGowin (1994) and Christine Boden (1998) show very convincingly that people with dementia do have something worthwhile to tell us.

Because I work with a different group of people, my approach necessarily differs from other forms of writing therapy. I will start, therefore, with an outline of the process by which poems such as *A Great Story* come into being. And what do these people have to say? Like all of us, they speak about families and their surroundings. But above all they show us how they feel about the experience of dementia. They express deep emotions that range over a wide spectrum. In many cases there is an awareness of the effects of the condition, although this is usually accompanied by bewilderment about the cause of these effects. And perhaps most interestingly, there is often a strong sense of self. We will look more closely at some of these expressions of emotion from the work before going on to discuss the problems arising from using words as a form of creative expression for people whose language skills are being eroded. The question also arises whether this activity qualifies for the title of 'therapy'. Is it therapeutic in nature? I can answer that only by reflecting on the reactions of the people involved in the process. The final justification for the work rests in what they have to say about their participation.

My twiddly bits

How do I go about collecting these words? Essentially I work in day centres, dementia-specific hostels and nursing homes or occasionally in a person's home. There I am available for anyone to talk with me. I work with people in varying stages of dementia most of whom can no longer write, although many can still read. So this is not creative writing in the strictest sense. Only the presence of an amanuensis makes it possible. One day May shook hands with me as her scribe. This simple act dispelled my earlier reservations. Using other people's words to create something new is deemed to be the worst crime in a writer's world. May went on to say: 'You're channelling this'. I felt reassured that this was not plagiarism. I now see myself as the channel or vessel through which these people's voices are made public.

Usually I write down the words long hand but with increasingly inventive abbreviations of my own. Unfortunately cassette recorders pose other problems. Not being at all selective they pick up all the background noise of music and clatter. They also pick up other voices, and so record the words of people who have not given permission for this to be done. Permission is essential and must lie initially with the speaker. Before recording any words I ask if I may do so. Sometimes that permission is refused. This happens only rarely, but the conversation still continues. It is simply not recorded. The family carer's permission is also sought before making any words public. In most cases I replace names with pseudonyms although some families have asked me to retain the real name.

Once I have typed out the transcript I search for themes running through the conversation. These phrases I copy and then arrange in a way that captures the essence of the words without changing any meaning by an inappropriate juxtaposition of phrases. This is where the writer's ear and sense for words becomes crucial. In this, as in all creative writing, I have found that the poems from each person have his or her distinctive voice, in spite of my intervention. These idiosyncratic voices help to convince me that the individual person-ness of each one is still present in spite of the damages caused by the dementia. It is this quality that I seek to preserve in the phrases selected for inclusion. On a subsequent visit I read the resulting poem to its owner for verification. Sometimes we discuss it. Sometimes they ask me to make changes. Responses have ranged from 'That's just what I wanted to say!' to 'Goodness, you think just like me!' and often 'Did I write a poem?'

The quality of listening is vital. It must be wholehearted, listening with the heart. Because of the emotional sensitivity that seems to develop in dementia, these people are acutely aware of any lapses in attention, any distractedness on my part. A passage in Hermann Hesse's *The Glass Bead Game* (1973) summed up for me this way of listening.

> His function was to arouse confidence and to be receptive, to listen patiently and lovingly, helping the imperfectly formed confession to take shape, inviting all that was dammed up or encrusted within each soul to flow and pour out. When it did, he received it and wrapped it in silence.
> (Hesse 1973, p.457)

Not that I 'wrap' their words in silence, but rather in acceptance and affection. There is in this work no element of reality orientation. For the

listener the speaker's world is reality. To listen empathetically requires a sus-
pension of judgement and the ability to enter into another's experience. This
places extreme strains on the listener. The requirements for a carer outlined
by Kitwood (1997, ch. 8) apply just as much to a writer working with people
with dementia. Above all it is essential that the writer should not neglect
caring for his or her own emotional well-being. I am thankful that John
Killick, in his early letters to me, insisted on this point. Just the title of his
recent article, 'Pathways through pain: a cautionary tale' (Killick 1999)
speaks movingly of his own experience. I have been fortunate from the
beginning to have the support of Judy Griffiths, who first suggested the
project to me. As a psychotherapist and grief counsellor working with
people with dementia, she has a special interest in the words I collect. She is
also there to 'hold the work' while I am holding the memories of the people I
talk with. We have regular supervision sessions when I share some of the
words collected. Very often Judy guides me towards unravelling possible
meanings behind them. She is also there, however, to help me resolve the
personal emotions aroused by spending hours talking so closely with people
with dementia.

My interest in such a project has its roots in my mother's move into a
dementia hostel. The words of the other residents fascinated me. At the same
time though, I wanted to understand more fully what my mother might be
going through. Having my own experience as a carer helps me in the
follow-up stage of the work, when I speak with family carers and seek their
permission for any public presentation of the words. To be able to say, 'I
know how you feel. I am there myself' certainly deepens our interaction.

The feeling of sorrow and sadness seems to come from right inside the heart

The 'ability to experience and express a range of emotions' is a major
component of a state of well-being (Kitwood and Bredin, 1992, p.281).
When we encourage people with dementia to speak freely, and when we
listen wholeheartedly and empathetically, we are invited to share the whole
gamut of their emotions. Perhaps, in fact, they may be more adept at experiencing and expressing feelings than their carers (Post 1995). The lessening
of social inhibitions which is typical in dementia may allow people to be
more conscious of their emotions and to voice them more openly. I have
found in fact not only that they have spoken freely about how they feel, but

also that they project these feelings so that I experience them as well. This tendency was pointed out to me in a supervision session and is commented on by Killick (1999, p.23).

Sometimes the words I collect remind me of the opening line by poet Gerard Manley Hopkins: 'I wake and feel the fell of dark, not day.'

In his early days in full-time care, Grant's words showed the same sense of despair. He, too, knew Hopkins' 'fell of dark'. Just 49 when I began working with him nine months before, Grant turned 50 a few months before he went into care. His condition had deteriorated markedly. Previously a very fluent speaker, he had shown an ongoing interest in the process of my work. As a feature writer for a local newspaper, a university lecturer and amateur comedian, his verbal and intellectual skills had been highly developed. Now he could hardly speak, walked with difficulty and appeared to have lost all concept of what I was doing. Nevertheless I recorded his words on my second visit to the nursing home.

What? – How? – Why?

Well, I've just gone.
I don't want…I don't know where I am
Fuck!
What's he doing?
What do you want to do?
He's got nothing.
I don't know.
I don't have anything to…
But how would it have come?
But I've never ever had…
So why do they do it to me?
Oh, come on! None…No.
They didn't come. Fuck!
I didn't even know what I was doing, was doing.
About that, that I don't know that I don't know.
What can I do? I'm not quite sure.

This poem is written just as it was spoken. Right at the beginning Grant indicated that he was confused, lost in his new surroundings. But might he not also be saying that the self he once recognized had gone, that he could no longer find the 'I' he knew before? Not only are Grant's words laden with questions stemming from a desperate attempt to understand what is happening to him, but also there is a potent metaphoric sense behind the questions and statements. While each relates appropriately to his present physical situation, the move to permanent care as well as the deterioration, they could as validly refer to a questioning of the meaning of life in its totality. We will look more closely at the language irregularities in the next section.

A passage written by Tim Brennan, a 55 year old in the United States, contains echoes of Grant's lament. Obviously written earlier in his progress through Alzheimer's, nevertheless these poignant thoughts express clearly that sense of loss.

> Often I find myself thinking about him. He was a person. He had an identity. The job he held was self-regulating and rewarding. He could do things, perhaps, many things.
>
> Now, it is so silly of me, I know, but sometimes, just for a brief moment, I like to think he is me – and I smile with the thought.

In a recent (1999) letter to me Tim wrote: 'I don't know this Tim. This person I am.' It is the same sensation as that within Grant's words: 'Well, I've just gone.'

In contrast to Grant's feelings of despair is this poem of his recorded five months earlier. As we sat in the sunshine at a local café, he told me of his thrill with learning at school. Grant loved comedy, playing the comedian himself in university revues and now as he spoke the accompanying mimicry created the image of an eager young puppy, begging for goodies.

Give Me More

> Wanting to know all of the things that were there.
> I want to watch this and see that
> and everyone's coming all over the place.
> Be the best in the school.
> That's what it was like.
> My mother was a teacher. I liked it!
> Give me more! Give me more! Give me more!
> I've done that one where is the next one?
> Can I come and have another?

> It was like that!
> There were all of these things you had to have.
> Like a young puppy.

These were the words of a man recalling the youthful adventure of discovery, the thrill of being 'the best', of chasing after knowledge and mastery. A long way from the despair of the 'modern Job' in the previous poem as he posed those unanswerable questions: What? – How? – Why? Together Grant's poems depict the rapid change that Alzheimer's brings.

For Rae the experience of Alzheimer's was also the 'fell of dark'. She was frightened of the dark as a child and so being in a dark place was an appropriate analogy for the fear Alzheimer's aroused in her.

> What is it if you take someone in a dark place
> and you leave them there for a very long time?
>
> ...
>
> Bit scary in the dark
> When I was in the dark I was frightened
> because the person knew I was frightened of the dark.
> So they had me on the short and curly.

A woman in her early sixties, Rae told me she was in a place to which she had been consigned by someone else, a place of punishment. Her words contained a strong sense of rhythm, that other component shared by poetry and music. At one moment she said:

> Otherwise the fear comes
> and the fear comes
> and then the fear comes more and more.

and again:

> You're floundering around in the dark
> getting more frightened
> and more frightened
> and more frightened.

No wordsmith could have crafted more powerful evocations of creeping terror. On the other hand Rae showed a determination to fight the condition as well as an impish sense of humour as she talked about how she planned to overcome this fear of the dark.

I'm going to learn the violin.
One of these days I will.
The Suzuki method.
You can give in or you can go nuts.

Later in the conversation she returned to the violin, laughing as she said:

I don't know what they're going to do
when I turn up with a fiddle.

May was often angry. She recognized her anger and the first day I recorded
our conversation she left no doubt as to how she felt.

Being Myself

I just want to be at home.
I have a right to this part
of the end of my life.
Yes, I am wringing my hands. I can't cope.
I have a right to a life of my own.
I am really very angry.
I just want to be at home – and be myself.
Do you have any ideas?

May was both unhappy and furious. She felt that this part of her life had been
taken from her. Which it had. Because of the dementia she could no longer
live in her own home, control her day as she pleased. A loner, she had to live
in close contact with fourteen others. She even had to share a bedroom with a
stranger. Some time later, when a new room-mate arrived, she took to locking
her out of their room. I could not help but feel it was an appropriate
expression of her deep feelings, a very natural reaction! But even more than
physical surroundings, May, like Grant and Tim, no longer recognized
aspects of herself. As she said later, she was getting 'tangled up'. She forgot
words, lost her train of thought. May had worked in a university and resented
this diminishment of her intellectual abilities. I felt it was significant that she
wanted 'to be at home' and 'be herself'. On one level she undoubtedly meant
that she wanted to be in her own surroundings again. But did she also mean
that she no longer felt at home with the changes that dementia had caused
within her being? That for her being 'at home' meant being the self she recognized, the self she had always been? During another conversation she said:

> It's like people coming and taking things from you.
> I feel as if my self is no longer any use.

While on one level she is referring to physical objects being removed from her room, I wondered whether this, too, had a symbolic meaning. Were the 'things' actually the abilities and memories which the disease was taking from her? Did going into Alzheimer's feel like a gradual robbing of the self? And to feel that her self, the essence of her being, was 'no longer any use' seemed the saddest feeling anyone could have.

Margaret's words on her first visit to a day-care centre left no doubt about her feeling of being lost. She spoke of the dementia without naming it.

> It has set me up the wrong way.

continuing:

> I've got no way.
> I've never had it before
> I've got to wait
> and see which way it goes.

To have no 'way' seemed an apt description of how a person with dementia loses control over their future. All those plans made years, months or days ago, must now be relinquished as the condition takes hold. For me her words created an image of someone standing some way into an expanse of scrub or bushland. No pathway is visible as yet. The figure can only stand and 'wait and see which way it goes.'

May also said that she must wait, without any certainty of what lay ahead.

> I just have to stand still in a way
> Which I'm not very happy about
> It's as if I'm waiting for something
> and I don't know why.

In residential care, is this sensation of waiting more pronounced because of the marked contrast between the residents, who usually sit or walk in quiet passivity, and the sometimes frenetic activity of staff and visitors? These latter have somewhere else to go, something important to do. The residents just have to wait; most of them do not know what they wait for or why. At times I have wondered what messages we send them through our body language, when there is a rush to serve meals, a sense of urgency about organizing an outing, or completing administrative tasks for the day. From my time spent observing in homes and hostels I am sure that people with dementia are highly sensitive to atmosphere and to the messages contained within our actions.

While many of these pieces are laden with questions, any attempt to interpret fully the words of someone with dementia must arouse more questions in the reader. Meaning lies on so many levels and I think it is the task of the writer to reveal these layers of meaning. We need to look within the words, unravel their possible connections and allusions, tease out the tangles and realize that these can be offered only as likely interpretations.

Some of the poems quoted above show obvious signs of language failure. Words are used incorrectly, sentence structure is confused. To what extent do these problems negate the possibility of significant verbal communication with people with dementia? We must first consider some typical linguistic problems and their effect on meaning.

I'm just blither-blathering

Neuroscientists are coming closer to understanding the mechanisms by which dementia affects the brain. It is clear, however, that various language functions are damaged. Probably the first problem which becomes apparent is a difficulty with word retrieval. In the early stages it is common for those I work with to berate themselves for being so stupid when they confuse words or cannot find the one they need. May recognized that she was 'tangled up'; Rae knew that she was 'scrambled'. While I have made no academic study of such language problems, years as a linguist and teacher of foreign languages, as well as my involvement in creative writing, mean that I am intrigued by the examples I find in the words I collect.

I have found that the mind tries to find the appropriate word in a number of ways. At times it offers a sense-related replacement. Irene always asks for a 'sniff-sniff'. The word 'handkerchief' seems to have disappeared all together, and yet her meaning is absolutely clear. Frequently the brain chooses a structurally related word having the same number of syllables and sound pattern. Several times Irene told me she was a 'loner'. One day, however, the connection must have slipped and she offered the replacement 'slower' – same syllable count and vowels, some difference in consonants. I am sure the word she wanted was 'loner', partly because of the earlier occurrences of the phrase. The 'slower' error occurred on only one occasion and it had some relevance as she was slowing down. Frequently the speaker recognizes that the chosen word is incorrect even offering alternatives. Speaking of her young days in a mining town, Annie talked of her father going to work in the mines. Each time she spoke of this she offered 'wine' and 'vine', showing by her questioning intonation that she knew very well that neither was the word she wanted. And each time, when I supplied 'mine', she agreed: 'Yes. They go down and down and down'. Was there any psychological significance in her inability to reproduce the word 'mine' while she retained so clearly the act of descent into the earth? Certainly throughout her conversation she revealed a strong memory of the dangers of going down in the lift to the tunnels below.

A common syntactical error is the confusion of personal pronouns. Often in conversation the speaker appears to jump from one person to another the way Grant does in his poem *What? – How? – Why?*

> What's he doing?
> What do you want to do?
> He's got nothing.
> I don't know.

It seems likely that in fact each statement and question applies to Grant himself. Or perhaps this is another example of two concurrent levels of meaning, encompassing his inability to understand what those around him were doing, both residents and visitors, as well as what was happening to himself.

In a similar way, the speaker may use an emotion or event from the past as a 'vehicle for expressing what she [or he] was feeling right then' (Griffiths 1995, p.4). In her grief work with people with dementia, Griffiths found that when one woman spoke of the death of her mother it indicated that she was feeling sad at that moment. Because the past event gave rise to the same feelings that the speaker was experiencing in the present, it could be used as a pointer to that emotion.

Another common confusion occurs with nouns indicating relationships. When someone says of a husband visiting his wife, 'He's come to collect his daughter', it may not be proof of how confused the speaker is, but rather a case of verbal substitution. Wives, daughters, sisters and aunts can appear in conversation in a disconcerting melange. With time I have learnt to relax about trying to track down absolute meaning. I wonder whether, in the long run, it really matters who did what. Instead I prefer to look for allusions, connections which might not normally be apparent and which might help me to understand the underlying emotion.

Talking about the effect of Alzheimer's upon her mind, Rae said: 'You get scrambled up in the dark'. Her thoughts were obviously confused. I had difficulty following her stories of an uncle who had played the violin for the Pope. I heard about violins at midnight, indigestion. But was it the Pope or the uncle who suffered? And why did the Pope hear the uncle's violin? My mind whirled with conflicting impressions and a conviction that she was very 'scrambled' indeed. Talking with her family, however, I discovered the truth of an uncle who was both a renowned violinist and a priest. Beneath the surface confusion lay a bedrock of facts. It provided me with a good lesson about not dismissing anything I heard without investigation.

Rae's words are a good example of the tendency of people with dementia to reconstruct reality (Hamilton-Smith 1996, p.3) by piecing together a story out of the otherwise fragmented facts available to them. The remnants of family history were cobbled together in a saving strategy which possibly helped her cope with the darkness.

Such confabulation occurs frequently and can be disconcerting for the listener. As I heard Clive's story of 'the last sword to sword fight' my mind was racing in an attempt to calculate his age and ascertain whether he could possibly have fought on horseback with swords. It seemed unlikely. Then I realized that he was actually telling me about the great waste of a life lost. Was this how he felt about ending his life with dementia? It was also a story which placed him at the centre of the action, a place he was no longer capable of holding. As he told me this story it seemed that the act of communicating was the most important element in the interchange. In such ways it seems that confabulation, too, may be a 'strategy for survival, a way of propping up one's threatened ego' (Crisp 1995, p.138).

Alongside the losses of language structure, however, there seems to be a freeing of imagery together with an increase in symbolism (Killick 1996, p.2). This gives rise to picturesque language that is well suited to a poetic medium. We have already seen Irene's expression 'up the ladder'. It appears as a refrain in the following poem in which Irene ponders on death.

Well Over the Top

I wonder when it exists when we fall down the ladder.
We seem to be the sort that'll be forever.
We seem to be just the same
How old would you be?

I'm bigger than you.
What have I got on the book?
I think I'm already at the top of the list.
I don't know exactly what the number is.
No matter what I'll still be there.
My sisters, they've gone from the list and time's passed.
I'm up to a long time.
But I know quite well I'm up the ladder,
but it's just the same.
I'm just the same as I was before.
Mine's well over the top.
I think at this stage of where I am now
it'll go one day –
but it doesn't upset me.
As far as I know
I'll always be somewhere around here.

Although she confuses the direction, is she going up or down the ladder, it is clear that going 'up/down the ladder' is her image for dying. And what an image it is! For me the immediate impression was of the childhood board game of Snakes and Ladders. Landing at the bottom of the ladder allowed you to move straight to the top of it, whereas landing on the head of a snake sent you slithering downwards. Perhaps this was Irene's mental image too, which could explain the confusion of going up or down the ladder. Combined with this however are intimations of Jacob's ladder, along which the angels passed from Heaven to earth; a sense of achievement, of getting to the top; a sense of passing from one sphere to another. Yet who can tell why she uses this expression? It has occurred in her language over a period of time, so was not a product of the moment. In this poem Irene uses other images for age which hint at approaching death: being at the top of the list, and having an age 'in the book'. Does this allude to the Book of Life and Death, in which perhaps the time of her death is already recorded? I find the imagery in such words refreshingly transparent. They allow us glimpses of layers of meaning which we will never be able to decipher clearly, but which lead us deeper into possibilities.

Irene's language is especially redolent with colourful images. On one visit after a longer absence she said: 'Here we are back in the same sock'. Her mother had 'a flock of children'. One of May's complaints was that doctors and staff had not 'learnt at my doorstep'. One day she said: 'Well, I'll leave you to do your twiddly bits', which seemed a perfect description of my role in producing these poems. I prefer to present these words in poetic form partly because of this symbolic language as well as the emotional content and innate sense of rhythm. While prose is the language of rational fact, poetry seems more suitable for expressing the heart's feelings.

You help some

Where does an activity such as this lie on the spectrum of dementia care? It is not strictly speaking reminiscence or autobiography. My interest is more in the inner world of the people I work with, their life now as they live with the condition. A lot has been written about the healing power of self-expression, whether it take the form of visual expression, song, dance or the written word. Poetry was seen as 'a natural medicine...like a homeopathic tincture' by poetic therapist, John Fox (1997, p.3) while the creative spirit within us all has been described as 'the medicine necessary for our own and planetary healing' (Cameron 1997, p.331).

To what extent is this work with the words of people with dementia healing for the speakers? Can it be therapeutic? As there is no known cure or remedy for dementia, perhaps no activity can rightly be named 'therapy'. It is unfortunate that, in these days when economic rationalism has become the determinant of policy, the only way that creative artists can market their work is by labelling it 'therapy'. Yet there is no doubt that the act of being heard and understood, of having your words valued, has a benefit for the speaker. This is where the value lies. It seems that 'the process is everything' (Killick 1998, p.107). The act of recounting our story is a powerful way of restoring well-being because our words and stories contain the essence of our self, the potency of 'our personal myths' (P. Miller 1994, p.9).

How much more restoring must it be for someone whose words are so often disregarded and dismissed by others, to be listened to, to have those words written down and held in a way that is beyond the scope of the speaker?

Music therapists Jungels and Belcher (1985, pp.134–137) tell the story of 66-year-old Hal, with whom they worked in a state mental hospital. Institutionalized since the age of 14, Hal was pronounced by doctors as '100 per cent uncommunicative' and 'mute'. When the music sessions developed into art sessions, Hal showed that he preferred to write words. Over time and with special activities, his withdrawal lessened and he began to converse with nurses and attendants. One day he told Jungels and Belcher: 'My cheeks are rosy anyway; I can't be dead!' (p.137).

In the words I have recorded I have heard many confirmations of the beneficial effect of the process. Charlie was almost incoherent and yet he loved to talk. He had great difficulty forming the appropriate words so that listening to him became guesswork and I had to ask often which word he meant. When I got it right he would say triumphantly: 'You've got it!' The transcripts of our conversations were so broken that the only way I could make a poem was to write about the conversation, including as many of his words as possible.

Poem for Two Voices

You speak so softly
Your words stumble into heaps about my ears
I lean to catch them
Piece them into sense.
'For'…'Four?'
I hold my fingers, count to four.
'No!'…'Before?'
'Yes.'…I do not know what came before, what followed.
'It's crit…crik…' 'Cricket?'
'No.'…'Critical?'
'Yes, you've got it!'…I'm glad, but not sure what it is.
'Smaller un…' 'Un?'
I can't get that word. Sometimes I feel helpless.'
'I do, too.'
'It's too late to put it…' Hand waves … 'The piano?'
'Yes.'…'Could you play something?'
'Now?'…'Yes.'
You stand, walk slow towards the piano, sit, feel for pedals
Fingers gather into curved bundles, tap at chords,
Right…left hand co-ordinate.
I am thrilled.
We talk of family. Four boys.
'All boys? No girls?'
'No, no girls. Mother was a girl.'
We laugh together.

'You help some…' 'Me?'
'Yes, you.'
'Does it help?'…'Oh, yes!'

The last three lines moved me deeply. When Charlie said: 'You help some', I made a point of asking if he really meant me, it is so easy to misinterpret. Again I checked that he meant it was my listening which helped. I was particularly touched by his statement that he, too, felt helpless. We were both struggling together for meaningful communication.

One day when May was especially furious, she said suddenly: 'It's lovely when someone like you comes along'. I asked her what it meant. 'It means peace'. This reply intrigued me. Did she mean that at least in our conversations she knew she was accepted, that what she said, thought and felt mattered, which in turn gave her a sense of well-being? Did the awareness of being heard release some of her stress and make her feel at ease?

Perhaps the most dramatic instance of change through the act of being heard and of telling your own story, came on a day when I was not recording the conversation. As I arrived in the hostel, Emmie was standing in the middle of the lounge room, her arms wrapped around her chest, eyes staring into the distance. Approaching her quietly I put my hand on her shoulder, saying: 'You look rather lost'.

'I've been lost ever since I came in here', she replied, and turned away.

A little later a staff carer brought her out to the patio where I was sitting with two or three residents. We were talking about childhood families. Gradually Emmie unwound. As she joined in the conversation she became more and more animated. We heard stories of her brothers and sisters, of their childhood escapades. It was an afternoon of laughter, sunshine and shared stories. After almost half an hour the group broke up and Emmie went back inside. Ten or fifteen minutes later she came out, stood before me, flung her arms wide and exclaimed: 'Here's the storyteller again!' Her whole body attitude expressed the difference that interchange had made. No longer tight and closed off from her surroundings, she was wide open and laughing. She had also remembered the episode.

This reaction to a time of sharing her story with interested listeners spoke more loudly than words about the benefit such an activity can have. To be heard and accepted as a worthwhile and unique human being is what we all seek in life. For the carers and family members it can also be a revelatory experience. While some family members are disturbed to see their loved one's dislocation confirmed in print, others appreciate the opportunity to contact the person they once knew so well. Within the institutional setting, carers tend to look at residents with new eyes after hearing words like Rae's as she describes being 'in the dark places'. For the writer working in this 'vanguard of a movement in dementia care' (Killick 1998, p.108) it is a rewarding experience accompanied by emotions ranging from light hilarity to deep distress. For me it is perhaps best encapsulated by May's words: 'You will be opened up a little'.

Acknowledgements

I wish to acknowledge and honour the people living with dementia who have allowed me to enter their worlds and record what they have to say. They have taught me a great deal. This is their story.

CHAPTER 4

The Importance of Singing with Elderly Patients

Alicia Ann Clair

Persons of all ages are generally fond of singing, but in some cultures when asked if they are willing to sing in the presence of others, there is great reluctance. Older adults are no exception to this, but many also reminisce about times growing up when everyone in the neighbourhood, or countryside, gathered frequently for an evening of singing. This singing, as it is described, represented community, a coming together of family and friends for a common purpose. It was a time to share experiences that contributed enjoyment and diversion from the trials of daily life. It gave opportunities to feel included and unconditionally accepted in the circle of people who provided mutual support no matter the circumstance.

These gatherings were the focus of recreational activities, and music was the centre. Conversations which describe them include comments about how singing was integral to many social events and how it was accessible to every one regardless of formal musical training. This singing was jubilant, vigorous and performed with little regard for how it sounded as a musical product. Descriptions of those who experienced it talk about how singing 'lifted the spirits', even when there was little over which to rejoice, and how it brought peace and warm feelings of comfort in addition to joy. In these outcomes, there was little concern for vocal excellence, and no one worried about how he or she sounded because every one was encouraged and supported as a participant. Actively making music together through singing provided a way to belong, to engage as part of a community where the very young to the very old gathered together to become one.

In some countries and in some cultures, people have moved from the use of singing as a form of active music-making for recreational purposes. Even so, there is often continued interest in singing as a pleasurable experience. When older persons are invited to sing, however, they often respond that they are fond of singing, but that they refrain from it because they do not have a 'good' voice. When asked to convey how that came about, they frequently say that they were told when they were young that they did not have a vocal quality that could contribute to a satisfactory musical, singing product. They were either discouraged from singing, or forcefully directed not to sing, on the basis of their poor vocal quality. These persons have gone through their lives denying themselves the enjoyment of singing with others, and perhaps even denying themselves the pleasures of singing when alone. From other older persons who are reluctant to sing, and who had reasonably good singing voices when younger, there are discussions of dissatisfactions with current vocal qualities due to ageing, and a reluctance to have their voices heard by others.

Singing for older persons, therefore, is regarded as meaningful, but there is resistance to participate in singing due to perceptions of vocal qualities. The music therapist who wishes to establish singing as a medium of intervention is faced with the challenge of encouraging and motivating people who have come to believe that their singing is poor, and who are reluctant for any one to hear more than their speaking voices. There is especial resistance to singing in the presence of a music therapist who is a musician first and foremost, and from whom individuals fear judgement and subsequent condemnation of their vocal quality. Therefore, music therapists struggle to establish a non-threatening environment that encourages singing, and dispels individuals' fears and anxieties of retribution for inadequate musical products. All this is prerequisite to the development of therapeutic outcomes with singing as the medium of intervention.

Perhaps there is so much concern about vocal quality because the voice, as a musical instrument, is so very personal. It is the voice that overtly demonstrates individuals' temperaments while it reveals their extraordinary, and not so extraordinary, qualities. It is the voice that provides the most observable and obvious indication of the human condition, including physical and emotional well-being. Therefore, it is important for individuals to have acceptable judgements of their vocal quality, and for these judgements to reflect the owner's worth through positive regard and appreciation. Very often, however, this does not happen, and individuals silence their voices as a result of comments that devalue their sounds as expressions of personal attributes and qualities. Instead, they believe their vocal sounds are poor musical products, and representations of themselves. Therefore, they consider their singing voices unsuitable for any setting or circumstance.

Rationale for singing as a form of therapeutic intervention

While there is little scientific research concerning the therapeutic benefits of singing, it is often observed that singing is integral to clinical applications of music in therapy across a wide range of population types and ages. Though the role of singing in music therapy is not clearly understood, it is indeed powerful in its influence. For the purposes of this chapter, it is postulated that singing in music therapy brings a point of human contact with other individuals, and this contact between individuals is meaningful and quite emotionally intimate. Therefore, singing is integrated into the human condition in some way and requires little to no cognitive processing to appreciate it. Consequently, singing is a viable intervention with those who have lost, or who did not develop, the capacities to cognitively process complex information. It is just as viable in situations where cognitive processing is contraindicated, unnecessary, or undesirable in the therapeutic process.

Perhaps the intimacy in singing connects with, or results from, individuals' experiences in which they were held, rocked, patted and sung to when they were in need of comfort. This may have occurred when they could not comprehend, or accept, the world around them, and also when they suffered emotional, physical or social alienations and traumas. The memories of particular events, or details of the events, in which such comfort was provided are often outside individuals' cognitive awareness. The positive, emotional feelings associated with them are relatively easy to retrieve, however, when singing is again provided. Therefore, positive responses to singing, and the desire to engage in singing, may have deep emotional ties for certain individuals throughout their lifetimes. For them, singing is interpreted as a source of comfort and relief from distress. It is this comfort function, and not the quality of the singing voice, that is essential to the beneficial outcomes.

The voice as an indication of the human condition

Contingent upon the role of singing in comfort is the power of the voice to reflect internal states. It is the voice that most quickly communicates the physical and emotional condition of the individual, with or without verbal content to augment the message. The full spectrum of the human condition is therefore evident in the sound qualities of the voice which range from indications of physical illness or emotional distress, to indications of physical well-being, contentment and even exuberance. While exact interpretation of an individual's vocal quality remains at issue until the full range of the particular individual's responses is known, there is clear and immediate indication of the response direction, and generally also its intensity.

The communication of internal states through the voice has its basis in the vocal anatomy and physiology. It is dependent upon the larynx, the sound-making mechanism in the throat, that is comprised of movable cartilage which change with musculature to alter the length and thickness of the vocal folds (Gauthier 1992). This function is contingent upon emotional disposition, physical tension and alignment of the body, including the position of the neck. These affect respiratory capacity and control, the amount and force of air through the vocal folds, and the shape and size of the resonating chamber. Collectively, these influence vocal sound quality (Gauthier 1992).

The physical tension and posture which influence vocal sounds are tied directly to emotional state. When the voice reflects depression or a low mood, the individual is likely to stand or sit with head down, and posture slumped. It is also likely that breathing is shallow, and located primarily in the upper chest. This results in vocal sounds that are poorly supported dia-phragmatically, with tones that are breathy, of short duration and pitched low, below the individual's optimum frequency. On the other hand, when the same individual is in a state of well-being, he or she is likely to have a well-aligned posture with head erect. Air is drawn deep into the chest cavity with proper diaphragmatic breathing. The vocal chamber is in its optimal position which allows for good resonance, and optimal frequency. The voice therefore sounds at a higher pitch, and utterances have longer durations than during the low mood condition. Vocal sounds in this condition may even have a certain 'singing' quality.

The voice, therefore, gives a good indication of how well an individual feels emotionally, physically and even spiritually. This indication is readily apparent, and everyone is familiar with times in their lives when they were asked, 'How are you?' and responded with, 'I'm fine'. Then to have as a coun-ter-response, 'You don't sound fine'. Chances are quite good that this coun-ter-response was accurate, even if the conversation occurred over the telephone without visual cues to provide information. The sound of the voice gives clear information that identifies the individual's positive or negative conditions that can either support or refute the individual's verbal content.

Because the voice indicates internal conditions of individuals, perhaps therapeutic interventions with the voice as a medium can function not only to alter negative or undesirable conditions, but also to maintain, and perhaps further develop, positive, desirable conditions. The music therapist, who is trained in a broad spectrum of music applications, must assess the condition of the individual, design a goal-directed intervention to remediate the needs, and/or develop a goal directed intervention designed to enhance the individual's condition.

The use of singing to influence mood positively

In the 1600s Richard Browne, an apothecary in London, wrote an essay which was published posthumously in 1729 on the therapeutic applications of music, particularly singing (Gibbons and Heller 1985). Browne claimed that singing could 'enliven the spirits' to remediate melancholia, a mood disorder now known as depression. He suggested that persons who were melancholic had simply to sing to improve their conditions, but it is now certain that appropriate health care is necessary for symptoms management.

Mood disorders, including depression, are complex and require a range of interventions for desirable management outcomes (American Psychiatric Association 1994) and while the incidence of depression in older adults is quite high, it is easily managed. This occurs with good medical care, adherence to appropriate pharmacological therapy, good nutrition, appropriate exercise, stress management, and involvement in meaningful activities. Such activities may comprise the therapeutic applications of music, including singing. While some research has shown that music combined with other interventions contributes to less depression (Hanser 1990), a study currently underway shows that active involvement in music-making contributes strongly to decreased depression (Tims 1999).

Generally, if persons are feeling depressed physically and emotionally, they are not willing, and may even feel unable to sing. Consequently, the mere suggestion of singing as a therapeutic intervention is often met with incredulity and scepticism. Admittedly, active participation in singing is very difficult in this circumstance, but the emission of vocal sounds that represent the individual's emotional and physical condition is possible, and is likely therapeutic. These vocal sounds are most often groans or moans that are initially short in duration and pitched rather low. Even so, the production of these sounds in a vocal intervention is an act of will that often requires encouragement, support and coaching from a qualified music therapist.

Singing interventions to lift mood can have several configurations. In one, the intervention begins after a very brief verbal introduction. It is followed immediately by the music therapist's sung vocal models supported with an improvised instrumental accompaniment suitable to the situation. Here the accompaniment is used to provide a non-threatening musical framework for the individual's vocal responses while it gives some structure to the experience. Initially, groans of short duration are encouraged by modelling, rather than verbal direction, in a call and response pattern. The therapist can alter the musical context to allow for direct imitation of the individual's vocal groan sounds, while changes in vocal pitch, loudness, rhythm, timbre and tempo, among others, are encouraged.

Such vocal sound production leads to two outcomes: a non-verbal expression of emotions which is important in the initial awareness of feelings, and physical stimulation which is conducive to deepened breathing, increased blood oxygenation and physical muscle tension release. Both of these outcomes function together to bring some temporary relief from symptoms. It is essential, though, for individuals to have appropriate medical care to assure best results from the overall treatment regimen. Singing must never substitute for medical care and pharmacological management, but can contribute significantly to the treatment process.

In this treatment context, it seems that vocal sound production can have best effects if it is used frequently, at least once and perhaps twice daily for 20 to 30 minutes. Assistance from a family or professional caregiver who is trained by the music therapist can encourage participation between scheduled music therapy sessions, or some individuals may possibly self-implement the groaning/singing applications. Such independent participation is unlikely, though, for those who have symptoms so serious that they are not motivated, or who feel unable to do anything.

Provided the singing intervention is effective, it is recommended that the music therapist provide a series of vocal sessions over a specified length of time to further develop singing processes that include melodic singing, melodic improvisation, lyric writing and others. It is also essential to provide support for those who are encouraged to explore how they feel physically and emotionally before and after their vocal experiences. It is imperative that the music therapist assess and evaluate outcomes regularly to determine whether changes in the intervention are indicated. Finally, as with all interventions, it is critical to determine when the therapeutic intervention has achieved its optimum outcomes, and the point of termination is at hand. Then, it is the responsibility of the music therapist to discontinue the intervention.

Singing as a form of active music-making to maintain wellness

Currently, active music-making as an approach to wellness in older persons was the focus of great attention by the United States popular media at the end of the 1990s. The sheer number of articles in major newspapers, and the inclusion of commentary on televised news programmes, indicate clearly the growing interest in getting and staying well through the later years of life. Statistics show that older persons are increasing in numbers, and as they age they are very interested in staying well to maintain their life quality (Winograd 1995a). One essential component of that life quality is to become and stay as functional as possible (Winograd 1995b).

A review of the literature shows that wellness is defined individually and includes components of physical, emotional and social functionality sufficient to maintain a good life quality. It is embodied in the absence of illness with low illness risk, maximum energy for daily living, enjoyment of daily life, continuous development of one's abilities, participation in supportive, satisfying relationships, and commitment to the common good (Schafer 1992, p.26). Therefore, older persons, even those who have chronic health conditions, can stay as well as possible.

The key ingredients for wellness include good nutrition, careful medical management, appropriate exercise, stress management, involvement in purposeful and meaningful activities, and responsibility for self-care (Gutt 1996). Balancing these components for each individual comprises a holistic approach to health and well-being. These components are therefore interactive, and a change in one affects the other.

Currently, a research study is underway to show the positive effects of active music-making on wellness in older adults. While this study is focused on keyboard playing, specifically the home organ, it has widespread implications for active music-making in other ways including singing. The preliminary outcomes of the study indicate that active music-making can decrease loneliness, decrease depression, and decrease anxiety, while it increases the level of growth hormone in older persons (Tims 1999).

Among others the components of this keyboard study are successful music playing, social participation in group lessons, wellness activities designed to manage stress, and the development of skills to provide independent access to active music playing which can fill unstructured time with meaningful, purposeful activity. Until further information is available regarding the benefits of the wellness activities designed for this study (Clair 1999), transfer to singing as an active form of music-making occurs through:

- singing favourite songs, either accompanied or unaccompanied

- involvement with others in social contexts where singing is the major focus, such as choirs and choruses

- singing to stimulate deep breathing and physical relaxation which are major components of most stress management interventions

- singing to lift moods

- singing to structure unscheduled time into meaningful, purposeful activity during the day or night.

Consequently, singing as a form of active music-making becomes, for those persons who enjoy it and desire to do it, a powerful component of wellness. It is important to note, however, that not all persons will find singing the most desirable form of music-making, but for those who do, it is likely as effective as playing a musical instrument.

For those who desire to sing as a component of their wellness programme, training with a skilled vocal instructor is essential, at least for a time. Such training is important because inappropriate and overuse of the voice can lead to injury, inordinate fatigue and the conclusion that singing is contradicted as a positive form of active music-making. Therefore, seeking an appropriately skilled vocal coach is a prerequisite to successful and ongoing engagement in a singing programme.

Access to vocal training, though important, can prove costly in terms of fees, proximity, transportation and other factors. It may also prove difficult to locate an instructor who is knowledgeable about older voices and is willing to work with older adults. Most choir directors are familiar with local vocal instructors and coaches, and can make referrals. These choir directors are also experienced coaches themselves, and they often have older singers in their choirs. Another resource is the choir conductor in the local school district who may want to provide training, and may even have an interest in a multigenerational singing programme such as the one described by Darrow,

Johnson and Ollenberger (1994). Here, older singers are incorporated into school vocal programmes as an integral part of the singing experience for both the senior singers and the youth singers. Outcomes have indicated a warm appreciation across the generations for both the older and the younger singers. The experience has provided pleasing musical and social opportunities for all.

If private instruction is desired, ready identification of private instructors who have experience and knowledge concerning the older voice is difficult. Many vocal instructors who have no prior experience with older singers may have a willing interest, however, if approached. They may become so committed that they carefully procure information in regard to physical and psychological needs of the older singers. Involvement with the first senior student may give some vocal instructors a new teaching direction which they find provides great satisfaction and appeal. Therefore, the requests by senior students for vocal training and instruction may lead to new developments in traditional studio work.

When a vocal trainer or instructor is located, it is important to communicate clearly a desire to engage in singing as an active form of music-making. It is also important to establish a time line for a series of lessons or sessions, with a definite fee structure, and clearly articulated goals. These goals provide guidance for the instruction, direction for the process, and a basis for outcomes evaluation. A series of regularly scheduled lessons will enhance commitment to a process that provides structure for positive experiences. These lessons also provide encouragement, support, and a good reason to sing daily.

While many older persons find contentment in singing at home alone, most also enjoy the social contexts of group singing. This can happen in a variety of venues including barbershop quartets and choruses, ethnic song and dance groups, choirs for religious services and functions, singing activities in civic groups, singing as an integral part of keyboard lessons, and others. Most of these opportunities can provide contact and close interaction with persons of various ages during the singing functions. They also have potential to lead to outside contact where people can meet to enjoy one another's company in non-musical activities. Singing, therefore, has the potential to build community for older persons who pursue it and desire contact and belonging with others.

Singing in palliative care

Munro (1984) defines palliative care as the abatement of troubling symptoms and the use of appropriate approaches that relieve distress. Palliative care further maximizes comfort for those for whom there is no expectation of recovery. It is administered in a wide range of situations where recuperation, restoration or rehabilitation is not possible. For the purposes of this chapter, palliative care focuses on two areas: hospice and late stage dementia.

Persons are deemed recipients of hospice care when they have reached the last weeks or days of life. In this time it is clear that death will come before long, and medical staff shift their focus from attempts to cure to efforts to remediate symptoms (Torrens 1995). There is great concern in hospice care to maintain quality of life; although that quality depends on individual preferences and opinions, it is generally comprised of physical, emotional, social and spiritual dimensions. The physical components focus on pain abatement, symptom management and discomfort control; it is possible to manage physical comfort readily with drugs. Emotional, social and spiritual comforts are, however, another matter.

Beyond the physical comfort of the patient, hospice care includes emotional support for the patient, the patient's family care provider, and other significant persons who visit regularly during hospice involvement. As part of the emotional support, there are opportunities for hospice staff and volunteers to talk through feelings with the patient alone, with the family, and with the constellation of patient, family and close friends. Though talking about feelings is indicated strongly as a way to move through the process of dying, it is often not all that is required. There are needs for both patients and others to have time together, to have some relief from emotional intensity, to structure some of the waiting time, to experience comfort, and to trust in a higher power that all will unfold in the very best way possible. Singing to and with hospice patients provides ways to meet these needs.

Early in the hospice situation, singing with the patient offers a way for all persons present to engage with one another. Often it is difficult to speak about certain issues, and singing provides desirable emotional contact and intimacy that gives comfort and alleviates fears without speaking. Even when spoken emotions and thoughts are desired, singing can give some time out from the emotional intensity associated with some verbal communications.

Often, the individual in hospice is desirous of ways to communicate verbally with family and friends, but the sadness inherent in the situation makes it difficult, if not impossible, for loved ones to tolerate such direct talk.

Therefore, music therapists have developed techniques of songwriting where hospice patients provide lyrics, and sometimes melodies also, to convey their thoughts and feelings to their loved ones in songs. Often, too, these hospice patients sing, or have the music therapist sing, while they record these composed songs on audio or videotape. Then, hospice patients are assured that their messages are left behind for loved ones to hear or see when the moment is not so emotionally volatile. They are satisfied that their messages can live on, and that the songs they have written convey their feelings for dear ones they will leave behind.

Besides hospice patients' active involvement in songwriting and music-making, there are opportunities to use singing as a way to decrease isolation, to elevate mood, and to provide ways to express spirituality. Though there is little research concerning the satisfaction of hospice patients with singing, two small-sample case studies contribute to the viability and efficacy of singing for persons in the last days of life. In the first study, Yonekura (1998) examined the effect of singing and physical touch provided by a music therapist on changes in voice quality of three individuals diagnosed with cancer and in hospice care. It was Yonekura's premise that the quality of the voice reflected the state of well-being of hospice patients, and that singing or singing combined with touch could influence it. Her results in cases studies of three individuals diagnosed with cancer showed that responses varied among participants; but, generally all three participants were responsive to singing, as indicated by higher spoken fundamental frequencies, increased ranges for spoken fundamental frequencies, and decreased spoken duration scores. Yonekura (1998) concluded that both singing and singing combined with touch had potential to influence changes in spoken voice qualities for hospice patients. She also indicated that these changes – increased spoken fundamental frequencies, increased ranges for fundamental frequencies and decreased spoken durations – were compatible with findings in the literature that associated these outcomes with positive feelings of happiness, enthusiasm, enjoyment and excitement. Therefore, it is likely that singing and singing combined with touch can increase hospice patients' positive responses through the last days of life.

In another case study, Koh (1998) examined the effect of singing on changes in facial expressions in case studies of three elderly individuals in hospice care. Koh provided her patients diagnosed with cancer a series of sessions individually in which she sang to them using their favourite songs. Analyses of videotapes determined facial behaviour repertoires. Generally, these behaviours included looking at the investigator, closing eyes, and dropping the jaw. All three subjects looked less, closed eyes more, and dropped their jaws more during the singing. A careful interpretation of these behaviours indicated these participants were more relaxed during the singing than during the pre- and post-baseline observations. Therefore, it was concluded that singing and singing with touch may affect responses of hospice patients which indicates increased relaxation and comfort.

The small-sample case studies conducted by Yonekura (1998) and Koh (1998) indicate that live singing has positive influences on patients in hospice care. In both studies, singing was done without accompaniment to assure accessibility to family and professional caregivers who do not have a musical background sufficient to provide their own accompaniments. Implications are that persons who simply sing songs familiar to and preferred by individual patients are likely to achieve a comfortable environment with positive experiences in hospice care.

Along with these outcomes, singing also affords something familiar at a time when the unknown is eminent, and when reminiscence is important to reach closure at the end of life. Songs associated with certain life periods can bring pleasant memories, and such memories can erupt in repeated enjoyment. Other songs may remind individuals of what is to come, and therefore trigger sadness and tears. Even so, these songs bring issues and feelings to conscience awareness to advance the potential for resolution of those unresolved feelings and issues in subsequent discussions. Such processes can lead to peace and comfort for all involved.

As hospice care proceeds to the last hours of life, singing can provide a context for the transition from life in this world to the next. Regardless of the beliefs held by all the people involved, this transition requires a 'letting go' by the family and significant others, and by the patient as well. Often, singing can offer a familiar framework that comforts in such time of loss, and empowers people to take some control in a situation where they cannot change the course of events. Family and significant others can engage in singing as a way to 'do something' for their loved one who is dying, while it affords them some comfort as well. It is recommended that the family gather around at the point of death to sing and to hold and caress their loved one. Moving into close proximity to put arms around, to hold hands, to smooth the brow or to touch in some other way is as important for family and significant others as it is for the dying person.

If the family desires some support with the singing, they may invite music therapists, music thanatologists, friends, clerics, nursing staff or others to provide it. Most of these persons incorporate the musical preferences of the family and the dying person into the singing. As the exception, music thanatologists sing medieval Latin chants, which they accompany on harp. Developed by Therese Schroeder-Sheker to allow dying persons to release from this world and to move to the next, music thanatologists are especially trained practitioners who work exclusively at the deathbed of those in their last hours of life (Schroeder-Sheker 1993).

Regardless of the approach and the music used, the objective for all singing at the point of death is a contribution to life quality until the mortal form exists no more. Consequently, singing that is appropriate to the situation is essential; it must not become a barrier to connections between family, significant others and the dying person. Therefore, great care is necessary to incorporate singing that contributes best to the situation and to the desires of the dying person, the family, and the people gathered to attend at the point of death.

Throughout hospice care, the purpose of singing is to contribute to life quality. Singing does so when it functions to create community as individuals share a common experience, to fill the waiting time meaningfully and purposefully, to give each person an emotional point of contact with one another and with the person who is dying, to give relief from the emotional strain of the dying process, and to afford some abatement from the emotional strain of impending loss. In addition, it functions to formulate positive and comforting memories for the survivors. Singing is truly natural, and beneficial to all involved throughout the hospice experience.

Singing in dementia care

Singing is integral to the life quality of those who are in progressive dementia and their caregivers. It functions to provide islands of arousal, awareness, familiarity, comfort, community and success like nothing else can. It is particularly valuable as an intervention because it is accessible to a wide array of individuals, since it has no prerequisites for prior musical skills or training, and it can include persons across cultures and socio-economic strata. It is also effective in severe, late stage dementia when responses to other stimuli are non-existent. Singing successfully engages individuals in meaningful, purposeful participation throughout the disease trajectory.

Benefits of singing go beyond the mere enjoyment of participation. Once engaged, singing naturally requires breathing deeply to produce phrases. As a result, it increases oxygenation and physical relaxation while it lifts mood. Furthermore, the success inherent in singing enhances individuals' dignity and worth. For those who are confused, singing provides comfort of the familiar, and an awareness of accomplishment when intellectual activity has become a way to failure, frustration and loss of control.

Early in the dementia process, singing is fully engaging for those who have always enjoyed it. Here, largely because of the disease process, inhibitions against singing may become less important, or at least less binding; individuals with dementia may become readily engaged in singing. In early stages, individuals are encouraged to implement singing participation themselves either alone or with others as active involvement in music. It is recommended that singing take the form of daily singing sessions at home, and if possible, involvement in community singing at church or in other settings. Singing sessions or lessons delivered by a music therapist, or an interested music professional, is further recommended. While such professional intervention is not critical to regular singing, it contributes support and encouragement while it incorporates a predictable schedule of meetings and practice sessions that add positively to daily routine and time structure. This is particularly important to compensate for losses when persons who have dementia must delete certain activities from daily participation due to the complex cognitive functions required to perform them. Active involvement in singing is certainly a positive and beneficial addition to daily routine when taking part in other components becomes inaccessible. In addition, daily engagement in singing contributes to elevated mood, and feelings of control and self-efficacy, along with physical benefits of decreased muscle tension.

Beginning early in progressive dementia, singing retains its value throughout the disease process. In middle stages, singing provides a way for persons to have experiences that are normal, where they can function as well as anyone else for a time. Here, as in the early stages, singing can have daily benefits, but it requires guidance and support from caregivers since individuals lose their abilities to self-implement. Individuals often spontaneously join in singing when exposed to it, and their continued participation is enhanced by eye contact and open facial expressions from those who lead singing experiences. A wide range of individuals can provide this singing leadership including music therapists along with professional and family caregivers. Participation durations last easily for 30 to 40 minutes with occasional cueing. For many, singing provides the longest durations of time where they are focused and clearly engaged in purposeful, meaningful activity.

It is recommended to include singing as part of the daily routine, and to schedule it prior to times when agitation, or apparent emotional distress, generally occur. Usually distress is associated with change which comes from such events as movement from one room to another, undressing and dressing, bathing and toileting, disruptions in routine, or changes in caregivers. Engagement in singing just prior to, and during, such times can function to facilitate physical relaxation through the processes of deep breathing required for singing phrases, release emotions through vocal expression, distract from apparent fear as it re-establishes trust, and provide a comfortable, familiar, predictable and structured experience that relieves the stress of change. Furthermore, singing for 10 to 15 minutes at various times throughout the day can restore the comfort necessary to alleviate, or at least diminish, distressing behaviours.

Singing familiar songs during middle stages of dementia is very successful in engaging participation because it provides experiences in the familiar that occur in a predictable structure provided by the music. Moreover, the structure and predictability of these familiar songs make it possible for persons to participate together with others. For many, who cannot function well enough cognitively to carry on conversations, or otherwise share in common encounters with others, this singing participation provides the only community they can experience. Likewise, it provides some of the only opportunities where family and other caregivers can interact functionally with their care-receivers who cannot follow the content of their verbal interactions, and who may no longer even recognize them. Singing in middle stages of dementia therefore provides a way to belong with others, and to contribute to normalized activities for those who have the disease and those who care for them.

As dementia progresses to late stages, people lose completely their abilities to perform activities of daily living. They also lose the abilities to verbalize and to move about. Consequently, they require round-the-clock care. At this point in the disease process, they are not able to function physically or socially, and typically show little or no response to external stimuli. Remaining responses are largely in the form of diminutive eye movements either with eyes open or closed, movement of the head to locate the sound source, movements of other body parts and, in some people, vocalizations.

While responsiveness is minimal at best, it remains essential to deliver programming that provides appropriate stimulation in order to maintain life
quality.

One research study shows that singing to individuals with late stage
dementia provides stimulation that elicits alert responses as indicated by
moving the head to locate the sound, eye blinking, eye movement under the
eye lid, movements in the hands or feet, or vocal responses (Clair 1996b). In
addition, this study showed, that reading the newspaper to individuals in late
stage dementia was also effective as a stimulus, but that singing was a more
powerful stimulus than reading as an influence over alert responses. The
clinical protocol used in this study also indicated different response styles
that were consistent for individuals over the entire series of four singing
sessions. In these styles some people were active responders, who may have
turned their heads, made vocal responses in apparent attempts to sing along,
or made some eye contact. Others were very passive responders. They gave
no apparent indication they knew the music therapist was present, and
appeared as if they were asleep. Careful observation revealed in these passive
responses such behaviours as eye movement under the closed lids, movement
of hands or toes, or opening eyes without eye contact.

The responses of the 28 participants in this study showed that singing
was an effective way to provide stimulation for persons in late stage dementia.
In addition, it demonstrated that responses can happen in a number of
different forms. Therefore, individuals who provide singing for persons in
late stage dementia must open their awareness to responses that may not
appear as expected, and a careful evaluation of the individual before, during,
and following singing is the best indication of effect.

In Clair's (1996b) study, care was taken to provide singing and reading
that were accessible to a wide range of caregivers. No accompaniment
instrument was used, songs familiar to most persons of the age range were
employed, information concerning preferred music for individuals was
gathered from family caregivers and friends whenever possible, and singing
was delivered in close proximity. In this simple context, singing successfully
evoked responses, and led to the conclusion that caregivers of various back-
grounds who are willing to sing are likely to evoke responses in persons with
late stage dementia. The most difficult task is to convince caregivers that the
quality of their voices is not important, but that their careful attention to the
individual and the delivery of familiar music are the critical features to elicit
responses with singing.

Music therapy clinical experience and research in late stage dementia has demonstrated singing as effective sensory stimulation in persons who can process no cognitive information, and who respond overtly to external stimulation in infinitesimal ways. These persons are still vulnerable to distressful circumstances, however, and it is important to provide calming influences prior to and during bathing, cleaning, physical examinations, medical procedures, dressing, and any other activity with which an individual has a history of distressful responses. Singing again has a viable role as a calming influence, and observation has shown less combativeness during and following singing, along with responses that appear serene.

Perhaps singing is so effective as a calming influence because people have associated it with comfort from the time they were small children. In their experiences, singing was paired with physical gestures of comfort, and never with aggression or hostility. At some level persons in late stage dementia know that singing is associated with tenderness, and that someone who is singing to them is not harmful or hurtful. They, therefore, are more likely to allow procedures without contentious behaviours. As a result, care-receivers and caregivers alike have less distress and physical trauma is avoided. Therefore, singing as a simple addition to the environment can improve the life quality for both care-receivers and their caregivers.

It is recommended that singing become an integral part of any programming provided for persons in late stage dementia. Scheduled singing for durations of 10–15 minutes, three or four times throughout the day is suggested. It is further recommended that care providers sing, at least for a few minutes, whenever they perform care procedures such as medication administration, bathing, clothes changing and other tasks. In singing they make contact with the care-receiver, and any resistance to their efforts are minimized, and often avoided.

Whenever singing is delivered in late stage dementia, it is likely to occur at bedside or chair side, due to the amount of support needed to maintain care standards for persons who are non-ambulatory and in the late stages of dementia. In any case, it is important to move into proximity appropriate for the individual while singing. This proximity varies among individuals, with some tolerating arm distance while others are quite receptive to hugs and caresses. It is also important to encourage spouses and family members to sing during their visits. While doing so, they may wish to position themselves so that they can embrace, hold, and perhaps rock, their care-receivers. Any demonstrative behaviours are left to the individual caregivers, but it is important to give them permission to use singing as a point of emotional intimacy, with or without physical contact with their loved ones.

It is through singing, then, that relationships are maintained, even when those care-receivers with dementia lose their abilities to initiate and recip- rocate interactions in usual ways. When all else fails, it is singing that holds care giving and care-receiving loved ones close in meaningful, non-verbal engagement. This closeness benefits caregivers who desire to maintain a con- nection with their care-receivers; although care-receivers cannot express it verbally, the connection with others through singing seems certain to enhance their life quality as well.

Singing in rehabilitation from stroke and Parkinson's disease

Singing has a long history in the rehabilitation of persons who have suffered strokes, and who have expressive aphasia. As part of this history, Melodic Intonation Therapy (MIT) was developed as a method to aid severely aphasic adults in the recovery of abilities to encode thoughts into meaningful units of verbal communication (Sparks and Holland 1976). The method was based on a series of clinical studies that used sung phrases to represent speech inflections and finger-tapped rhythms to cue prosody. The method fades the singing and maintains the tapping as patients go on to speak the short, previously sung phrases.

MIT has had some success over the years, and is recently under adaptation by Corene Hurt Thaut, music therapist at Poudre Valley Hospital, Fort Collins, Colorado (C.H. Thaut 1999). Ms Thaut, who is a member of the neurologic rehabilitation team at the Center for Biomedical Research in Music at Colorado State University, works in conjunction with speech pathologists in the rehabilitation of persons with expressive aphasia due to strokes or traumatic brain injury. She has recently developed a technique from the MIT method which uses longer phrases than the original version and adds guitar accompaniment. The instrumental accompaniment helps to set the rhythm for the phrases, while the longer phrases allow for response latency and establish syllabic rhythm that sets the timing for responses. This clinical adaptation is based on theories of rhythmic cueing derived from basic research conducted by Dr Michael Thaut and his associates at the Center for Biomedical Research in Music, Colorado State University, Fort Collins. Here, external rhythm organizes rhythmic responses, such as that required for ambulation and other body movements (M. Thaut 1999b).

Outcomes of Corene Thaut's adaptations of the MIT method in clinical applications have yielded exceptional results, and clinical research to examine these outcomes is in process. An established clinical protocol for widespread use is sure to follow.

Additional clinical research in music therapy has employed singing interventions in rehabilitation programmes for persons with stroke and traumatic brain injury. Dr Nicki Cohen, currently at Texas Women's University, Denton has pursued a line of inquiry that indicates positive benefits of singing. Cohen has concluded that singing leads to improved speech because it encompasses the essential elements of correct speech production (Cohen 1992, 1994, 1995a, 1995b). Furthermore, singing develops breath support, vocal projection and expanded vocal range, all of which are essential to speech intelligibility (Cohen and Masse 1993).

Cohen's (1995b) treatment protocol includes breathing instruction, vocal exercises and familiar song-singing. Furthermore, she encourages home practice for which she provides tapes with pre-recorded breathing and vocal exercises to guide the practice.

While speech rehabilitation for stroke patients has a long history, efforts to remediate speech problems in persons diagnosed with Parkinson's disease is rather new. Until recently, persons with Parkinson's disease were not referred for speech treatment, although 75 per cent of them have speech problems, because they were considered to have no potential for rehabilitation (Ramig *et al.* 1994).

In an effort to meet the physiological and emotional needs of Parkinson patients for speech, Eri Haneishi (1999) developed a Music Therapy Voice Treatment Programme (MTVP) at the University of Kansas, Lawrence. She tested the programme with four females over a series of twelve to fourteen 60-minute sessions held once weekly. She encouraged vocal/singing practice between the sessions.

Haneishi examined auditory recordings of her programme participants for vocal intensity, speech intelligibility, maximum duration of sustained vowel phonation, maximum vocal range, vocal fundamental frequency and vocal fundamental frequency variability. She further assessed their mood. Statistically significant increases were found in vocal intensity and speech intelligibility, with increases in fundamental frequency that approached statistical significance. Mood significantly increased when measurement scores before and after each session were compared. No significant increases were found in the analyses of tapes recorded before and after each session in vocal intensity, fundamental frequency, and fundamental frequency variability. Haneishi concluded this lack of change was likely a function of fatigue.

Haneishi considered Cohen's (1995b) applications in the development of her protocol for Parkinson's disease patients. Haneishi structured her protocol around conversation, warm-up exercises, vocal exercises, preferred song-singing, vowel sounds, exercises to practice for the coming week and closing conversation. Adjustments were made for individuals according to their respective vocal capacities and disease process stages.

As Haneishi continues to develop and test her protocol, preliminary results are outstanding. Her contributions are certain to guide the practice applications for speech recovery and maintenance in persons who have Parkinson's disease.

Conclusion

The importance of singing for older persons is largely overlooked in many cultures. It seems that singing has found its role as a way to fill time, an activity that has little importance when compared with others. Clinical outcomes in music therapy refute this role and indicate singing as a viable, efficacious medium in the engagement of older adults in appropriate applications to promote and maintain their life quality.

Singing can meet the functional needs of older adults through a broad range of abilities and disabilities. Consequently, involvement in singing as a form of active music-making is important to the health and well-being of older adults. Even when individuals are limited in their vocal ranges and abilities, active singing can promote health through its physiological, psychological and social benefits. Perhaps the greatest obstacle to older persons' singing is the cultural bias which discourages it, or even forbids it. Until such time that cultural endorsements of wellness include singing as a form of active music-making for all, regardless of age and expertise, participation is encouraged and supported by those who understand its value. Music therapists and other professionals must consider the benefits of singing for wellness interventions that include older adults, as well as persons who are younger. In these efforts, it is important to train the older singer to avoid injury and to promote the best possible outcomes.

For those older persons who have diagnoses of progressive diseases, singing can serve as an integral part of the treatment process. When these individuals progress to the point that palliative care is required, singing gives essential comfort and human contact. It further contributes to symptom management. Persons who become so debilitated from age and/or disease that they can no longer function, can still respond to singing. It provides a way to belong with others until mortal life has passed, and while it brings benefits to the care-receiver it provides the point of contact for the caregiver as well.

Whether involvement in singing includes active participation or passive listening, singing has great potential as a contributor to wellness and to treatment in therapeutic interventions for older adults. Singing provides connections with personal histories and contact with others in the present while it acknowledges personal identity and dignity. It is certainly powerful in its influence, and is accessible to all who desire it as a means to comfort and satisfaction. Consequently, singing is an important consideration in the life quality of older adults, and efforts to develop further tested music therapy applications and protocols are strongly indicated.

CHAPTER 5

The Problem of Agitation in Elderly People and the Potential Benefit of Music Therapy

Annemiek Vink

'Madame, when are you finally taking me home?' Questions like these are often to be heard on geriatric nursing home wards. For caregivers of demented elderly people it is a stressful task to remain calm when the same question is repeated over and over again, especially when there are other tasks that need to be done. Repetitive sentences or questions are very common in demented elderly people. As many as 90 per cent of elderly patients with dementing illness demonstrate problem behaviours, which may range from repetitive verbalizations and wandering to verbal and physical aggression towards themselves and others (Davis, Buckwalter and Burgio 1997).

Most of the demented elderly people in our society live at home. When the disease progresses, they become more restless, they suffer from disturbed sleep and may start to act aggressively towards the family caregivers. Often, these behavioural problems are too difficult to cope with for the family relatives and nursing home placement becomes inevitable. Although it is recognized that these problem behaviours are a major burden for both caregivers and demented elderly people themselves, relatively little research has been done to understand these behaviours and find interventions to manage them effectively. In the clinical literature, problematic disruptive behaviours are often referred to as agitation. In this chapter the causes of agitation will be discussed and the potential benefit of music therapy to reduce these problematic behaviours.

The problem of agitation in demented elderly people was first described by Cohen-Mansfield and Billig in 1986. Since that time agitation has been defined as an inappropriate verbal, vocal or motor activity that is not judged by an outside observer to result directly from the needs or confusion of the agitated individual. To understand more of the prevalence of agitated behaviours, Cohen-Mansfield, Marx and Rosenthal (1989) undertook an observational study in a nursing home. The Cohen-Mansfield Agitation Inventory was developed, an observational checklist listing 29 of the most troublesome behaviours that form the cluster of agitated behaviours (see Table 5.1). All items were gathered based on information from nursing home staff.

Table 5.1 Agitation related behaviours in dementia

Cursing or verbal aggression	Kicking	Inappropriate robing/disrobing	Repetitious sentences
Hitting	Scratching	Performing repetitious mannerisms	Complaining
Grabbing	Eating/drinking inappropriate substances	Trying to get to a different place	Negativism
Tearing things	Hurting oneself or others	Handling things inappropriately	Making strange noises
Pushing	Intentional falling	Throwing things	Screaming
Biting	Physical sexual advances	General restlessness	Hiding things
Spitting	Pacing	Constant requests for attention	Hoarding things

Source: Cohen-Mansfield Agitation Inventory (Cohen-Mansfield, Marx and Rosenthal 1989)

In a total of 408 nursing home residents the frequency of agitated behaviours was observed. It was found that 93 per cent of the 408 residents demonstrated one or more agitated behaviours at least once a week, with a mean number of 9.3 agitated behaviours weekly. The behaviours most often found to occur were making strange noises, requests for attention, repetitious mannerisms, picking at or inappropriate handling of things, strange movements and pacing.

The most remarkable finding in the study was that behaviours did not occur separately, but rather there seemed to be a pattern of coexisting behaviours. Within the group of agitated behaviours, three clusters of such co-occurring behaviours have been differentiated.

The first group of aggressive behaviours includes behaviours such as hitting, kicking, pushing, grabbing and cursing. The second group of physically non-aggressive behaviours consists of behaviours such as pacing, general restlessness, inappropriate robing or disrobing and repetitious mannerisms. Last, the group of verbally agitated behaviours includes behaviours such as screaming, complaining, negativism and constant requests for attention.

Ever since agitation in demented elderly people was first described, the literature concerning agitation has been diverse. Agitation is a broad term that includes a variety of problematic behaviours. Nevertheless, over the years it has been shown that observers can rate these behaviours with great accuracy. Although the definitions of agitation vary from time to time, they all include behaviours such as anxiety, tension, irritability, restlessness, wandering, physical and verbal aggression, confusion and disturbed sleep (Brotons and Pickett-Cooper 1996). Agitated behaviour is always socially inappropriate behaviour and may be manifested in three ways; as abusive or aggressive behaviour toward oneself or others, as appropriate behaviour but with an inappropriate frequency or as inappropriate according to social standards, such as putting on too many clothes on a warm day (Cohen-Mansfield *et al.* 1989).

What causes agitation in dementia?

To understand more of the causes of agitation, insight is needed in the processes present in dementia-related diseases. The most characteristic feature of dementia is the progressive decline of cognitive functions. The period between the onset of the first symptoms of dementia and the last phase is often described in three phases. During these phases there are a variety of changes that a demented person goes through. In the early phase of dementia, personality changes may occur, the patient becomes easily irritated and there is reduced interest in social and daily activities. Memory deficit becomes increasingly apparent, which is often manifested in restlessness. At the end of the first phase, the patient can no longer function without some form of assistance and nursing home placement becomes inevitable. As the disease progresses to the middle phase of dementia, problematic behaviours increase such as screaming, wandering and physical and verbal aggression. Paranoid delusions and hallucinations may also appear. A typical form of a delusion which is often heard is that the spouse is seen as being an impostor. In this middle phase of dementia patients also start to forget the name of their spouses and become largely unaware of the major events in their lives. It is becoming increasingly more difficult for the demented persons to express their needs verbally. In the latest phase of dementia all cognitive and verbal abilities are gone. Most of the time, the patient is capable only of making mere sounds without the ability to speak (aphasia). When all other functioning decreases, the patient becomes bedridden and in the end will die (Reisberg *et al.* 1982).

Agitation is clearly linked to these three phases of dementia and may occur in all three phases. The dominance of the type of agitation differs depending on the disease progression. The presence of agitation has been found to be related to a more rapid annual decline of cognitive functions (Brown University 1995). Cohen-Mansfield, Marx and Rosenthal (1990) described the relation between feelings of agitation in relation to the rate of cognitive decline in dementia more precisely. The results indicated that agitation was more prevalent among cognitively impaired than among cognitively intact residents, with the highest levels of agitation being exhibited by those in the middle phase of dementia with moderate levels of cognitive impairment. However, agitation was also quite prevalent among cognitively intact residents. Manifestations of agitation appeared to differ between cognitively intact and cognitively impaired residents. Residents with severe cognitive impairment tended to exhibit more aggressive and physically non-aggressive behaviours where cognitively intact individuals manifested more verbally agitated behaviours. All forms of agitation seemed to decrease in the later stages, when all functioning further decreases. Verbal and hiding or hoarding behaviour seemed to be more prevalent among cognitive intact residents, and is less associated with cognitive functioning.

Cognitive decline has been found to be a major determinant for the presence of agitation. Disturbed sleep patterns, which are thought to be the result of a decrease in cognitive functioning, are also related to the presence of agitation. An overall lack of hours of sleep and disruptions of sleep have been found to be related to the presence of agitated behaviours during the day (Cohen-Mansfield and Marx 1990). A typical pattern which is seen with demented elderly people is that agitated behaviours increase at night, after the onset of the late afternoon, which has aptly been described as 'sundowning' agitation (Hopkins, Rindlisbacher and Grant 1992).

Finally, it is important to consider psychosocial determinants of agitation. The amount of activity and distraction offered to the residents is related to the degree at which agitated behaviours are manifested. Cohen-Mansfield (1992) reported the striking finding in a 3-month observational study of 24 residents, that they were unoccupied 63 per cent of the time observations were made and were highly agitated, indicating that boredom is a major predictor of agitation. Overall, the patients manifested a greater amount of agitated behaviours when they were unoccupied and less agitation when involved in music therapy and other structured or social activities such as the visit of family relatives.

There is no single cause for agitated behaviours to occur. It is important to consider constantly with each resident and each behaviour what may be the cause of the agitation. For some there may be organic causes while with others the agitated behaviour may be an expression of discomfort. Cohen-Mansfield (1996) described one of the residents in a Jewish nursing home as being constantly aggressive during bathing times. When it was understood that the aggression was possibly caused by the association with showers in the concentration camps during the Second World War, other solutions could be sought. From the last example it can be seen how important observations are in the understanding of agitated behaviour. People with dementia have progressively more difficulties in expressing themselves verbally. Careful observations should therefore be made to interpret the agitated behaviour. Music therapy, with its non-verbal qualities, is especially suitable for these patients whose verbal abilities are declining (Aldridge 1992, 1993a).

The effect of music therapy in reducing agitation

It is only recently that there has been more attention for the need to find interventions to reduce agitation. Management of behavioural symptoms in patients with dementia is essential to improve the quality of life for the patients and their caregivers. Aggressive elderly people may cause harm to themselves and to others, although it must be understood that the aggression is an act of fear rather than intentional aggression. The more that agitated behaviours occur, the more that agitated elderly people require supervision. This means an increase in the numbers of nursing home staff for which often no financial sources are available. An alternative is to find other approaches to reduce agitated behaviours. Pharmacological approaches are effective to treat some of the behaviours. Symptoms that are known to be effectively treated with drugs include physical and verbal agitation, depression and various psychotic symptoms. Other symptoms such as wandering, hiding and hoarding behaviour and stealing are not treatable with medicine and require other approaches (Ahmed 1995).

The use of drugs in handling behavioural syndromes is often not preferable as there are many side-effects, such as drug–drug interactions, dizziness, increased risk of falling and adverse effects such as an increase in agitation. Neuroleptic agents which are often offered in the treatment of agitation are known to cause motor agitation and increase wandering behaviour. Also the dosage is difficult to determine due to the slower metabolism of elderly people.

General advice is to investigate first whether non-pharmacological interventions can bring about changes in the behaviour before medication is started. Prinsley (1986) recommended music therapy for geriatric care in that it reduces the individual prescription of tranquillizing medication, reduces the use of hypnotics on the hospital ward and helps overall rehabilitation. Several studies indicate that through non-pharmacological interventions agitation can be relieved, through music therapy, for example.

Wandering behaviour

One of the behaviours that can typically be found in demented elderly people is wandering behaviour. Often, patients are seen in the nursing homes pacing up and down the corridor in a restless manner. Doors have to be constantly locked as it too often happens that the wanderers fall and injure themselves when they enter unknown areas. Wandering behaviour is part of the cluster of problem behaviours that make up anxious or agitated behaviour. Lucero et al. (1993) tried to describe wandering behaviour of institutionalized patients with Alzheimer's disease in their natural environment. It occurs mostly with patients in middle and late stage dementia. The need for interventions is, according to Lucero et al. (1993), greatest during unstructured periods of the day. Often, physical restraints are used to prevent wandering behaviour but rather than preventing agitation, the use of physical restraints actually increases the amount of agitation (Werner et al. 1989).

Groene (1993) researched the effect of music therapy in reducing wandering behaviour with 30 Alzheimer's disease patients (aged 60–91) in the late and severe stages of dementia. For the baseline measurements, the wandering behaviour of each participant was recorded for a minimum of three days, between 2.00 p.m. and 5.30 p.m. The subjects were randomly assigned to either a mostly music condition (e.g. five music sessions and two reading sessions) or to mostly reading sessions (e.g. five reading sessions and two music sessions). Each subject received each day of the week, for a maximum of 15 minutes, alternated sessions of individual reading and individualized music therapy.

Music therapy sessions consisted of listening to music, playing instruments, singing, and movement or dance. Live music activities were incorporated in each session. Reading sessions consisted of the therapist reading aloud to the client or the patients themselves read aloud. Both activities were, when possible, adjusted to personal preferences. Seating proximity behaviour, the amount the patient remained seated or stayed in the room, was recorded on videotape and was used as an estimate for a possible decrease in wandering. Also the Mini-Mental State Examination was administered before and after the sessions to record changes in cognitive functioning. There were no significant changes in MMSE scores for both groups, from pre- to post-treatment measurements. The amount of time wandering subjects remained seated was longer for music sessions, regardless of whether they participated in the mostly music or reading sessions. Wandering in general outside the sessions did not decrease.

Fitzgerald-Cloutier (1993) also compared the effect of music therapy to reading sessions in their respective success in decreasing wandering behaviour in a female Alzheimer's patient (aged 81 years). The subject showed very frustrated behaviour and the music therapist tried singing with her to help her remain seated. After 20 singing sessions, the therapist read to the patient in an effort to compare the degree of attentiveness. Reading and singing sessions were timed according to length of time the patient stayed seated. Both music therapy and reading sessions redirected her from wandering, but the total time she remained seated for the music therapy sessions was double compared to the reading sessions (214.3 minutes versus 99.1 minutes). It was noted that the length of time she remained seated for music therapy increased consistently, whereas the time she sat during reading was more sporadic. Several studies have shown that wandering behaviour decreases due to music therapeutic intervention (Clendaniel and Fleishell

1989; Fitzgerald-Cloutier 1993; Groene 1993; Olderog-Millard and Smith 1989).

Agitation during bathing

Behavioural problems are very time consuming in the care for these patients. A simple task, such as bathing or toileting, can take hours due to aggression and non-cooperation. Although many results have been reported about the burden on caregivers of demented elderly people, relatively little research has been directed towards effective methods of managing behavioural symptoms of demented patients. Management of behavioural symptoms in patients with dementia is essential to improve the quality of life for the patients and their caregivers.

Two studies have described how music can contribute to a decrease of aggressive behaviour during bathing. Clark, Lipe and Bilbrey (1998) studied the effect of tape-recorded music during bathing episodes with 18 residents with severe Alzheimer's disease. For a period of ten weeks, the residents' preferred music was played and alternated with a period of ten weeks where no music was played. Results indicated that during the music period decreases occurred for twelve of the fifteen observed agitated behaviours. The five most frequent recorded behaviours were yelling, abusive language, hitting, verbal resistance and physical resistance. Decreases were significant for the total number of aggressive behaviours and for hitting as separate behaviour. In these studies a direct effect of music was found as well as an indirect effect on the caretakers. Caregivers noted that during the music episodes, the mood of the residents was improved, they were smiling more and were more co-operative, making the bathing task more pleasurable for the caregivers.

A similar study has been conducted by Thomas, Heitman and Alexander (1997). A total of fourteen patients with Alzheimer's disease were observed during bathing times. All were diagnosed as middle stage dementia. A music tape was recorded with help from family members. Typical musical selections included the music of Glenn Miller and Beethoven's Moonlight Sonata. Regretfully, the study design did not involve an extended intervention period. Only on three occasions was music played with each resident, where in contrast caregivers received a three-week training programme on observing and selecting music. No significant reductions were found for verbally agitated behaviours, physically non-aggressive behaviours and hiding or hoarding behaviours. Significant reductions were found for aggressive behaviours as was the case in the previously described study.

Agitation during bathing is often the result of sudden changes of environment, such as going to the bathing room or to the dining room. Any major environmental changes may cause agitation as the place looks unfamiliar. Even such small changes as moving a chair can cause agitated behaviours such as aggression.

Mealtime agitation

An environmental change is also apparent when residents are brought to the dining room and often residents become highly agitated. Typical for the community rooms in a nursing home is the large amount of background noise. Several researchers have studied if background music can contribute to a less disturbing nursing environment. Goddaer and Abraham (1994) investigated if playing tape-recorded music in the dining room could reduce the general noise level. Through decreasing the noise level, it was expected that agitated behaviours would decrease. Twenty-nine demented residents participated in a four-week music programme. In the first week, no music was played in the dining room and baseline observations of the prevalence of agitated behaviours were made. In the second week relaxing music was introduced in the dining room. The music was selected on the basis of slow tempi and additional music was selected from New Age recordings. In the third week no music was played, to be later reintroduced in the fourth week. Subjects were observed with a dichotomous version of the Cohen-Mansfield Agitation Inventory (see Table 5.1). Significant reductions were observed on the cumulative incidence of the total observed agitated behaviours (63.4%), as well as the incidence of physically non-aggressive behaviours (56.3 %) and verbally agitated behaviours (74.5%). No reductions were observed in hiding/hoarding behaviours and aggressive behaviours. The presence of agitation followed the distinct pattern of the study design. Agitation decreased from the first week to the second week when the relaxing music was introduced (54%), increased in the third week (38.4% = control period) and decreased in the fourth week (43% = music period) when again music was played during dinner. From this study it can be concluded that music indirectly affects feelings of agitation through reducing the general noise level.

Similar results have been reported by Denney (1997). She replicated Goddaer and Abraham's (1994) study with a few modifications. In this study, nine demented residents participated and instead of daily observations, weekly recordings were made of the presence of agitated behaviours. The residents were studied during lunchtimes, while light classical music was played with a tempo of between 50 and 70 beats per minute. Also in this study the presence of agitation followed the typical pattern of the study design. In the first and third week no background music was presented. In the second week agitated behaviours decreased with 46 per cent compared to the first week. During the third week agitated behaviours increased but were still 8 per cent below the baseline measurements. In the fourth week agitated behaviours decreased compared to the baseline with 37 per cent. Verbally agitated behaviours were affected the most through the music intervention.

From the above described studies it is clear that agitation decreases as a result of slow relaxing music. Is this the type of music that should be used to obtain the best results?

Ragneskog *et al.* (1996b) studied whether the observed effects depended on the type of music played and if food intake increased as a result of music listening. Three types of music were used. First, soothing music, then old popular Swedish songs from the 1920s and 1930s (songs that the patients would typically know from their youth) and last, contemporary pop music. Each type of music was played in the dining room for two weeks, while patients were coming in to have their dinner. Between the musical periods there were one week intervals in which no music was played. The reactions of the patients to the three different types of music were videotaped. Four out of five patients spent more time at dinner during the music periods than in the control periods. The study showed that all the patients who were having dinner were affected by music, particularly by soothing music. Individual responses that were observed during the study were that one of the typically restless patients became unusually calm, whereas another ate more than usual. Significant improvements in symptoms of irritability, fear and depressed mood were seen when music was played at meals compared to the control period without music. Soothing music was found to have the most beneficial effect. These benefits appeared to persist right through the control period. The study concluded that indeed slow relaxing music can improve symptoms associated with dementia and stimulates elderly residents into eating more.

Clair and Bernstein (1994) studied whether there is a possible decrease in agitation linked to a particular music style. Their study aim was to see if the use of background music is a viable method to decrease agitated behaviours. Twenty-eight severely demented residents participated in this study. This study questioned if there was a possible difference between sedative music (music for mellow minds) and stimulative music (popular big band music) in the effect to reduce the amount of agitated behaviours compared to a situation in which no music was present. Also it was studied if the effect of music depended on the time of day: morning, noon and afternoon.

The morning and afternoon music was played in the day room. At noon music was played during mealtime. Music was played for an entire day, five days a week for a period of eight weeks alternated with a control condition in which no music was present. Observations were recorded three times a day for a total of ten days per condition. In this study there was no significant change observed in the amount of agitated behaviours as a result of the music intervention, although a trend was found that sedative music was more likely to decrease the amount of agitated behaviours than no music or stimulative background music. Overall, it can be concluded that slow music is effective to reduce agitation when presented as background music. Clair and Bernstein (1994) on the other hand explain the lack of change in their study as a possible result of the fact that the same music was used for all subjects, instead of individualized music. Could individualized music perhaps be more effective in reducing agitation?

The effect of individualized music on feelings of agitation

Gerdner and Swanson (1993) studied the effect of individualized music sessions in reducing agitation. Five female patients (age range 70–99), all diagnosed with probable Alzheimer's disease (score <21 on MMSE), participated in this study. All subjects were confused and agitated. The content of the music therapy sessions was based on musical preferences as was reported by close family members on the Modified Hartsock Music Preference Questionnaire. Each patient received five daily individual sessions from 3.30 p.m. to 4.00 p.m. with tape-recorded music of their preference. The presence of agitation was evaluated with a modified Cohen-Mansfield Agitation Scale and with the Mini-Mental State Examination for cognitive function on pre- and post-treatment measurements.

Observation data were collected for one week previous to the sessions. During the following week, when music sessions started, the observations continued from 3.30 p.m. to 5.00 p.m. The session itself was held from 3.30 p.m. to 4.00 p.m. The results were reported individually. Overall, feelings of agitation decreased with more than 50 per cent after the sessions compared to the baseline measurements. One patient showed no significant decrease, because already in the baseline agitation scores were very low and there was no information available about the role music played in her life. For other patients it was indicated that music was very important during their lives. The importance of music may be a significant influence on the subjects' response. The degree of change greatly varied among the five patients. For the researchers this was an indication that music sessions should be individualized to obtain the best effect. Casby and Holm (1994) studied the effect of individualized music with demented elderly people. In particular they studied whether listening to music is an effective means in reducing repetitive vocal outlets among three Alzheimer's disease patients. They observed the residents while they were listening on a headphone set to classical music (Pachelbel's Canon in D) and music of their own preference. The frequency of vocal outlets were compared to a normal situation in which no music is listened to. Both listening to classical music as to the music of their own preference reduced the amount of vocal outlets significantly.

The effect of active music therapy on feelings of agitation

In all the previous studies effects were reported of tape-recorded music in reducing agitation. Both background music and individualized music have been found effective in reducing agitation. Many music therapists question if there are differences between the effect of tape-recorded music versus active involvement in music activities with demented elderly people. Brotons and Pickett-Cooper (1996) studied if active music therapy in small groups could also influence the patients' feelings of agitation. Also studied was whether different responses were the result of a difference in musical background of the patients. Twenty patients participated in this study, seventeen female and three male, with a medium age of 82 (age range 70–96). All patients were diagnosed with probable Alzheimer's disease and all were in the middle phase of dementia with moderate to severe impairment. Fourteen patients (70%) were given medication to control behavioural disturbances.

At the start of the study they all scored above 8 on the Agitation Behaviour Scale, an observational five-point scale checklist measuring seven problem behaviours: pacing, hand wringing, inability to sit or lie still, rapid speech, increased level of psychomotor activity, crying, and repetitive verbalizations of distress. Agitation in this study was defined as the presence of hyperactivity, physical restlessness and not being able to sit still. The caregivers measured agitation in the morning hours, just before the session started, and observations were made after the session had ended for another 20 minutes. All sessions took place in the afternoon. During the sessions the patients were videotaped for posthoc observation. It was investigated if there were noticeable changes in medication, agitation and if musical background influenced the responses on the music activities. Musical background was scored as either if someone enjoys music and has been involved in an ensemble for more than three years, or if one enjoys music and has had three or more years of musical instruction. The patients were divided in groups of three or four participants and received twice a week music sessions of 20 minutes, for a total of five sessions. Each session included at least one of the following activities: singing, playing instruments, dance/movement, musical games and composition/improvisation. The order in which these activities were presented was constant throughout all the sessions. The session started with a greeting song, then there was a dance or movement activity, a musical game, composition and improvisation tasks, and then playing along with pre-recorded songs. The session ended with singing one or two songs as a group. The results showed that there was no effect of musical background and there was a significant change in agitated behaviours. Specific behaviours that significantly decreased, in comparison with the baseline observations, were pacing and crying. There were not enough data to note changes in medication. The changes were consistent when pre- and post-session measurements were compared. A continuous decrease in agitated behaviour was observed when post-treatment scores were compared to the scores from before the session. But there was inconsistency from session to session. According to the researchers, the nature of the subjects and their unpredictable behaviour was the cause for this inconsistency. Most probably, the small number of sessions could also have produced this inconsistency.

Conclusion

In this chapter the effects of music therapy have been described in an effort to show that music therapy is a viable non-pharmacological intervention to reduce agitation in demented elderly people. Most studies indicate a clear decrease in agitated or related behaviours through music intervention.

Specific behaviours that are part of the cluster of agitated behaviours that have been found to decrease are vocally disruptive behaviour, hitting, wandering, crying and pacing and an increase in hours of sleep (see Table 5.2).

It can been questioned whether there is a difference between the responses of demented elderly people when they passively listen to music or when they actively participate in the music-making in active music therapy. Both background music and individualized music listening seem to be effective in reducing agitation. When background music is used, careful considerations should be made. Music may evoke negative feelings or memories which may lead to an increase in agitation. At all times a skilled music therapist should be consulted to advise in music selection.

Table 5.2 Specific agitation-related behaviour changes brought about by musical interventions	
Vocally disruptive behaviour	Casby and Holm 1994; Denney 1997; Thomas *et al.* 1997
Hitting	Clark *et al.* 1998
Wandering	Clendaniel and Fleishell 1989; Fitzgerald-Cloutier 1993; Groene 1993; Olderog-Millard and Smith 1989
Crying and pacing	Brotons and Pickett-Cooper 1996
Increase in hours of sleep	Hanser 1990; Lindenmuth *et al.* 1992

From the studies reviewed, it is relatively unknown whether group therapy is as effective as individualized treatment. Most often music therapy with demented elderly people consists of small group sessions as it is in practice too expensive to serve all patients individually. Only one of the studies reviewed involved group activities. In the study of Brotons and Pickett-Cooper (1996) active music therapy in small groups was successful in reducing agitated behaviour. It is not known from this study if all musical activities equally attributed to the decrease in agitation or if one type of activity is particularly effective. Gerdner and Swanson (1993) state that for a positive effect of music therapy, it is important to individualize music adjusted to musical preferences. On the other hand it is equally well possible within small group sessions to adjust to individual musical preferences by choosing songs and music of the 1920s and 1930s that are typically known for the group members. Also the group members could be selected on the basis of a shared musical interest.

The number of people suffering from dementia is rapidly increasing and so too are the workload increases for caretaking staff. Caregiver burden is strongly associated with the presence of agitation, mainly with physical aggression and repetitive questions or statements (Victoroff, Mack and Nielson 1998). In several reports it has been informally described that not only the patient benefits from the music sessions but their caregivers as well. Brotons and Pickett-Cooper (1996) describe that the decrease in agitation, as a result of music therapy intervention, carried over to the rest of the afternoon and that even in the evening periods there was still a noticeable decrease. Nurses stated that patients came back more calmer, more co-operative, more responsive and a lot nicer. Olderog-Millard and Smith (1989) also found in their study on the effects of music therapy an unexpected beneficial effect on the caretaking staff. During the five-week course of the study, nursing staff often reported that music seemed to calm the patients and to increase their orientation to the present. Staff members also expressed surprise and pleasure at seeing the patients singing and were especially surprised to see the more regressed patients, those who rarely spoke, singing. Nurses stated that during the music sessions they could complete charting duties as interruptions decreased. The researchers concluded that seeing these patients participate in singing and hearing live music on the unit could possibly help to decrease staff burnout.

Improvement in research designs

The current state in music therapy research involving the study of agitation in dementia is promising. Music has a significant effect in reducing agitated behaviours but many aspects are still unknown. More researches are needed to be able to understand better the effect of music with demented elderly people. The studies described in this chapter were all relatively small in terms of the number of residents studied. Another gap in the study designs is the lack of control for other factors that could have been equally responsible for a decrease in agitation, such as medication. Only in one study were changes in medication recorded, yet there were insufficient data to conclude whether a decrease in agitation resulted from the music activities. Also other factors could have accounted for a decrease in agitation, such as the visit of a relative, as Cohen-Mansfield (1992) observed.

In the music therapy studies previously discussed, often the population of subjects is described as diagnosed with probable Alzheimer's disease. Others have described the effect of music on patients who are severely demented. The latter findings are more descriptive for this particular disease stage, but are difficult to generalize to other patients. In most studies differentiation within the population of patients has not taken place, with MMSE scores ranging from 0 to 21, indicating a large variety of functioning within the patient group. A more apparent effect of music therapy can be described when one differentiates more within the patient population and when one includes more patient characteristics other than age and sex, but for example also patients' characteristics which are thought to be related to the presence of agitation and to cognitive decline. Various patient characteristics can contribute to an overall decline during the research period. When one uses only group totals on evaluation measures in the analyses, as is often the case, the scores of patients who deteriorate faster or have a different symptom presentation will influence the total outcomes. In the study of Gerdner and Swanson (1993) the individual differences in scores were very apparent. When, in future researches, the client population is better defined and more attention is given to possible intervening variables, clearer recommendations can be made for each stage of the disease course for music therapists working in practice with demented elderly people.

How does music work?

Another question that is important to be researched more thoroughly is why music has the ability to reduce agitation in demented elderly people. The first and foremost obvious reason is that music induces relaxation and reduces stress-related hormones, such as cortisol. Although much has been written on the topic of the relaxing qualities of music, relatively little is known with this particular patient group. Others have referred to the Progressively Lowered Stress Threshold Model (Hall and Buckwalter 1987). Following this model, the threshold for experiencing stress lowers as a result of declining cognitive and social skills. According to Hall and Buckwalter (1987), maximum functional levels can be achieved not by challenging to regain lost functions but by supporting the losses. Following this model, the music activities should fit the abilities of the individual to obtain optimal participation. Both ideas should be pursued more to be able to understand better the effect of music on demented elderly people.

Coda

The future for music therapy with demented elderly people is promising. Nursing home care for institutionalized demented elderly people has gone through many changes over the years. Earlier descriptions on care for demented people were mostly based on a medical model. Patients were given basic care and medicine to cope with the secondary symptoms resulting from dementia. During the 1980s and 1990s, a transition was seen from a 'disease'-oriented approach towards a focus on the social and psychological consequences of dementia (Droës 1998). Instead of trying to slow cognitive deterioration, care approaches are needed that stimulate present abilities, focus on improving the quality of life of the residents and reduce problematic behaviours associated with dementia. Music therapy clearly serves all these goals.

Acknowledgements

This study is supported by grants from the Dutch Alzheimer Foundation (Alzheimer Nederland), Triodos Foundation, Fund Music Therapy of Buma Stemra and the Rens Holle Foundation.

CHAPTER 6

A Survey of Music Therapy Practice with Elderly People in the Netherlands

Annemiek Vink

Music therapy as a profession is relatively new in general health care. In the Netherlands, since the 1950s and 1960s, the first music therapists started out to work with psychiatric and mentally retarded clients. Today, most music therapists in the Netherlands are still working with these client populations. The introduction of the music therapist in the nursing home is of more recent date, although especially with this client population the positive effect of music has been long recognized.

Many studies have described the beneficial effects of music therapy upon dementia. Music therapy has been found to improve social and cognitive skills and as a result of music therapy intervention problematic behaviours, such as wandering and repetitive vocal outlets, have been found to decrease (Casby and Holme 1994; Groene 1993; Olderog-Millard and Smith 1989; Pollack and Namazi 1992; Pickett and Moore 1991).

A large proportion of the music therapy literature involves the scientific study of the effect of music therapy with elderly people. In most studies, the intervention consisted of individualized receptive music therapy whereas in practice generally music therapists use a varied range of methods, such as improvisational music. To what extent active music therapy is used in psychogeriatric practice is unknown. Relatively few studies give insight in the actual practice of music therapists working with demented elderly people. Questions are asked regarding what choices does a music therapist make when for instance working with demented patients? Which goals are set when working in psychogeriatric practice and does one work indeed mostly with individual patients as the literature suggests? With these questions in mind a survey study has been held among Dutch music therapists working in this field.

How many music therapists work in psychogeriatric practice?

Survey studies conducted in Canada and the United States show that the number of jobs increases in all sectors in health care on a yearly basis. The Canadian Association for Music Therapy (CAMT 1996) reported that in 1996, 31 new positions were created compared to 7 positions lost. Results were based on the analysis of 114 questionnaires; 52 music therapists (46%) indicated that they were working with Alzheimer's disease patients.

The American Music Therapy Association (AMTA 1998) reported similar results based on 2034 surveys. In 1998 68 new positions were created versus 20 positions lost. It was indicated by 697 music therapists that they were working in a geriatric facility, a geriatric psychiatric unit or in a nursing home. Unfortunately, few statements were made about the respective increase for each specialization on a yearly basis. Allison (1992) interviewed all (!) 45 music therapists in Australia and stated that most music therapists (43.1%) were working with elderly people.

To learn more about the current proportion of music therapists working in psychogeriatric care in Europe, several music therapy associations were contacted. Music therapy associations in Germany, Britain, Denmark and Finland were asked if they also had similar survey results. Although all indicated the usefulness of these statistics, none of the associations knew how many music therapists were working in their respective countries.

In the Netherlands, it has been estimated that in total 291 music therapists are currently employed in general health care (Neijmeijer, Wijgert and Hutschemaekers 1996). The total number of creative therapists has been estimated at 1040. In all, it was expected that 49 music therapists were working in psychogeriatrics, the third largest clinical population after the mentally handicapped and psychiatric populations. Estimates in this report were based on membership of the Dutch Association for Creative Therapy (Nederlandse Vereniging voor Kreatieve Therapie). Not all music therapists are actually members of this association, so it was expected that the actual number of music therapists working in psychogeriatric care would be higher.

To answer the question how many music therapists are currently employed in geriatric care, a questionnaire was sent out in 1998 to 247 nursing homes in the Netherlands. Of the 247 nursing homes, 153 returned the questionnaire (61.9%). Analysis revealed that over 95 per cent of the residents on the psychogeriatric care unit of the nursing home are demented. In 32 (22.9%) of the psychogeriatric nursing homes, music therapy is offered to demented residents and in total 33 music therapists are employed in these nursing homes. In 39 (25.5%) nursing homes where no music therapist is employed, the use of music in other activities was mentioned, mostly during activity therapy and recreational activities. The number of nursing homes has increased to 300. When the data are extrapolated to this number of 300 homes, the estimated number of music therapists working in psychogeriatrics would amount to 60 in total. This corresponded to the number found when the names reported in this survey were combined with several other existing address lists. In total the addresses of 60 music therapists working in psychogeriatric care in the Netherlands were collected. When it was known how many music therapists were working in psychogeriatrics in the Netherlands, a survey was sent out to learn more of the work carried out in practice.

Description of the instrument and subjects

A 57-item questionnaire was developed for the purpose of gaining more insight in music therapy practice in psychogeriatric care in the Netherlands. The first section of the questionnaire started with general aspects of the profession, such as training and job-related experience. Also questions were included to learn which sources music therapists use to educate themselves further on recent developments in music therapy. An extensive body of the literature music therapy students in the Netherlands read are Dutch or German language publications. To what extent professional therapists also use foreign literature and theories developed abroad is relatively unknown.

In the second and third section of the questionnaire, mostly open-ended questions were used, since this was the first attempt to survey music therapists in psychogeriatrics and no information was available to define fixed categories. The second section included questions about music therapy in psychogeriatric care in general. As most of the residents are demented and an estimated 60–70 per cent of demented elderly patients suffer from Alzheimer's disease, the third section of the questionnaire involved the work of the music therapist working with Alzheimer's disease patients.

Aspects addressed in the second and third sections were:

- Whether therapists worked with group or with individual treatment?
- What is the average duration of the intervention?
- Whether therapists worked with active or receptive music therapy?
- How are active and receptive music therapy used in practice in terms of content, instruments used and musical repertoire used?

The questionnaire was reviewed by two music therapists to see if all questions were easily understood and to see if all questions were unambiguously stated. A pilot study was held among five music therapists, to see if items needed to be adjusted.

Subjects

The revised questionnaire was mailed to 55 music therapists and a reminder letter was sent out to increase the response rate. A total of 33 (60%) question-naires were returned and 32 (58%) were suitable for data-analysis. Of these responders 7 were male (21.9%) and 25 female (78.1%). The average age of the responders was 38 (age range: 26–57). The music therapist in psycho-geriatrics has on average 6.5 years of experience (range: 0.5 to 25 years) and works an average of 76 hours per month (range: 10–160 hours per month). Twenty music therapists indicated that they were employed in one nursing home, five in two nursing homes and two music therapists were employed in three homes at the same time. In the next sections of this chapter, the most important survey outcomes will be reported.

Theoretical background of the music therapists

In the Netherlands, there are several music therapy training programmes lasting four years, which are placed within the regular educational system in the Netherlands (Smeijsters 1993).

Of the responders, nineteen (59%) were educated at one of the four music therapy training programmes which are allied with the colleges of higher vocational education (Hogeschool) in Enschede, Utrecht, Nijmegen and Sittard. Four music therapists (13%) graduated from one of the two ortho(ped)agogic music training programmes available in the Netherlands, in Alkmaar and Maastricht. Two music therapists (6%) were trained at the

'Wervel' in Zeist, a music therapy school where music therapy is taught on an anthroposophic basis. The other seven (22%) responders were trained elsewhere, for example studying at a conservatoire and following courses in music therapy. None was trained abroad or had followed advanced courses in a foreign country.

In the Netherlands there are no postgraduate studies for music therapy. In the survey, questions were included to learn more of the ways music therapists educate themselves, after they have graduated from music therapy training. Table 6.1 lists the several sources, ranging from reading music therapy journals to talking with other colleagues. In separate questions the therapists were asked if they knew the source of information and how often they used the source of information, which was answered on a six-point scale ranging from never (1) to always (6).

Talking with other colleagues is the option which was most known to the responders and is most frequently used when informing themselves about recent developments in music therapy. The *Dutch Magazine for Creative Therapies* is the second most popular source to refer to. This magazine is received automatically by registered members of the Dutch Association for Creative Therapies (NVKT). Relatively unknown and read sources are *The Soloist*, the Dutch journal for self-employed music therapists, and the journal *Music Therapy Perspectives*. A possible reason is that *The Soloist* is relatively new in the Netherlands and also in psychogeriatrics there are no music therapists working on a self-employed basis. *Music Therapy Perspectives* is not available through Dutch libraries, which could explain its low score.

The largest proportion of the responders reported that they seldom made use of any of the mentioned sources. The main reason is probably that most journals are hard to find in libraries; however, easily accessible sources, like the Internet, are seldom used too. More surprising is that most foreign journals, like the *Journal of Music Therapy*, are also relatively unknown, which seems to confirm that mostly local information is used. Possibly, responders have confused the *Journal of Music Therapy* with *Music Therapy*, which is also not available in Dutch libraries. In general, the possible variety of resources mentioned are not used on a regular basis.

Questions were also asked about which theoretical views the clinician uses in practice. During music therapy training in the Netherlands, various theoretical approaches are taught to the students. A typical theoretical orientation that has been developed in the Netherlands is the analogous process model by Smeijsters (1995), in which it is assumed that pathological

Table 6.1 Use of sources providing information on recent developments in music therapy

Do you know this source of information? How often do you use this source of information?	% Yes	% No	Mean	Std dev.
Talking with other colleagues	31 (96.9%)	1 (3.1%)	4.06	1.24
Dutch Magazine for Creative Therapies (Tijdschrift voor Kreatieve Therapie)	30 (93.8%)	2 (6.2%)	3.38	1.70
Attending music therapy conferences	30 (93.8%)	2 (6.2%)	2.59	0.91
Internet	24 (75%)	8 (25%)	1.62	0.91
Professional meetings	23 (71.9%)	9 (28.1%)	2.25	0.98
Music Therapy	16 (50%)	16 (50%)	1.56	0.88
Musiktherapeutische Umschau	15 (46.9%)	17 (53.1%)	1.53	0.76
Journal of Music Therapy	9 (28.1%)	23 (71.9%)	1.31	0.69
Journal of British Music Therapy	8 (25%)	24 (75%)	1.38	0.87
Arts in Psychotherapy	8 (25%)	24 (75%)	1.28	0.68
Zeitschrift fur Musik-, Tanz, und Kunsttherapie	5 (15.6%)	27 (84.4%)	1.12	0.42
The Soloist (De Solist, a Dutch journal for self-employed music therapists)	2 (6.2%)	30 (93.8%)	1.03	0.18
Music Therapy Perspectives	1 (3.1%)	31 (96.9%)	1.09	0.39

n = 32

processes are reflected in musical processes. The following short descriptions of the various theoretical approaches were given to the music therapists and they were asked to indicate according to which background(s) they work with in psychogeriatric care (see Table 6.2).

In general it was expected that in line with other specializations in health care, most music therapists would be eclectic in their approach depending on the clients' characteristics. This was indeed the case. Only two of the music therapists surveyed followed one theoretical orientation in their work in psychogeriatrics following the creative process model. On average, music therapists selected three alternatives to describe their theoretical orientation

---

Table 6.2 Theoretical orientations in music therapy

Psychoanalytical music therapy
Through the unconscious exploring of music, by listening to music or through improvisation, associations can be stimulated. The transference relationship, in which the client in a symbolic way experiences suppressed situations again, can help someone to release tensions and can provide new insights.

Behaviouristic music therapy
Through the use of music as a stimulus, relaxation is induced in the listener, as a counterbalance for one's fears. Also music can be used as a reinforcer for positive behaviours.

Humanistic music therapy
Through unconditional acceptance of the client's (musical) expression and through a warm and honest approach, the client opens up in progressive steps. Clients discover their true personality and can make more realistic choices for a more desired future life.

Communicative music therapy
During musical improvisation it is studied how the client interacts with others and how this is expressed in music. The analogy between the concrete musical, the desired social behaviour and the client's experiences become apparent in a playful situation and this gives clients the opportunity to experiment with themselves and in interaction with others.

Analogous process model
In this model it is assumed that musical behaviours are in a sense a reflection of clients' daily lives, including their psychopathology. Through the use of musical methods it is possible to (positively) influence the clients' overall behaviours and their experiences.

Creative process model
A process in which clients can use creative processes (such as music) to release themselves from rigid patterns in relation to their direct environment by searching for their own personal composition, which is adjusted to their own desires.

Source: Derived from the original Dutch version of N. van Nieuwenhuizen and M. Broersen (1998)

in their work. In Table 6.3 the frequencies are reported for each of the theoretical orientations. The least used option was psychoanalytical music therapy and the most popular orientation was humanistic therapy. There was no consistent pattern to be found in the way combinations of theoretical orientations were reported. Further it seemed that age was a predictor of theoretical orientation. The modal age of the sample was 35. Although there were not many changes related to age, music therapists older than 35 more often reported that they worked according to psychoanalytical music therapy.

Table 6.3 Theoretical orientations in the work in psychogeriatrics

	Age <35	Age >35	Total N
Psychoanalytical music therapy	2	7	9 (29.0%)
Behaviouristic music therapy	6	8	14 (45.2%)
Humanistic music therapy	11	7	19 (61.3%)
Communicative music therapy	6	9	15 (48.4%)
Analogous process model	8	6	14 (45.2%)
Creative process model	5	9	14 (45.2%)
n = 31			

Furthermore, it was asked how theoretical orientations were translated to music therapy practice. Music therapists indicated in behaviouristic music therapy that music is used to structure the clients' experiences, which releases fear. Other music therapists stated that music stimulates memories which influence the clients' behaviour. Also it was stated that through the use of music, positive behaviours can be stimulated, such as relaxation.

Most reactions were given in relation to humanistic music therapy: unconditional acceptance of clients and their musical expressions serves to provide a sense of safety and comfort basic to human well-being. Others indicated that the chosen orientations did best reflect their own ideas on music therapy or that were trained as such. In respect to the analogous process model it was stated that with demented elderly people with declining verbal abilities, the musical expression is indicative of the client's feelings. In regard to the creative process model, music therapists stated that clients are stimulated to get close to their own experiences and learn to express their inner selves. About communicative music therapy it was mentioned that through musical improvisation non-verbal communication patterns can be stimulated, especially when the verbal abilities are gone.

In general the following music therapy techniques were reported in the work in psychogeriatrics but were generally unrelated to the theoretical orientation: musical improvisation, singing or playing along with familiar music, interactive musical games, using themes from daily life in musical play, reminiscence activities, following or leading in musical play and imitating musical behaviours. It seemed too difficult for the respondants to describe music therapy methods according to theoretical orientations as most music therapists work intuitively and are eclectic in their approach.

Drieschner and Pioch (1998) questioned if this implicit knowledge can be explicated. They asked if there are implicit rules in the choices that music therapists make when adapting music therapy methods to certain clinical populations. Music therapists from four health-care sectors were interviewed in this study ranging from adult psychiatry, child psychiatry, care for elderly people and care for mentally handicapped people. The data of thirty music therapists were analysed. Therapists provided significantly more structure in music therapy with elderly people and children compared to music therapy with adults. The music itself and the interaction between the patient and the musical material was considered most important by the music therapists working with elderly people. Drieschner and Pioch (1998) write that music therapists found it very difficult to distinguish between different methods in their practice. Many music therapists seem implicitly to develop a personal style based on intuition.

Music therapy with psychogeriatric residents

Most nursing homes have separate somatic and psychogeriatric wards, where respectively residents reside who have primarily physical or psychiatric problems. Most (over 95 per cent) of the residents who stay on a psycho-geriatric unit are demented. Music therapists indicated in the survey that patients are primarily referred to music therapy when they have social problems, when they are agitated or display passive behaviour. Further indications are emotional problems and the residents' affinity with music.

Most of the residents who are referred to music therapy are demented. The following disease groups were reported in order of significance: Alzheimer's disease, multi-infarct dementia or vascular dementia, Parkinsonian dementia and Huntington disease. Other major diseases that were reported included CVA, Korsakoff, acquired brain damage and depression.

In the literature it has been stated that the best time for music therapy intervention is in the late afternoon before the peak level of agitation is reached (Gerdner and Swanson 1993). Other researchers (Goddaer and Abraham 1994; Ragneskog et al. 1996b) mentioned that at lunchtime the residents are often restless, which indicates that this would be the best time of day for music therapy. It was questioned in the survey if the music therapist also had a preference for a time of day to conduct music therapy. Most indicated that they had no special preference for a time of day at which they believed music therapy would have any other additional effects. When a preference was indicated it was for the morning hours, when residents are more awake, or at the beginning of the afternoon (see Table 6.4).

Table 6.4 Music therapists' preferences for a time of day for music therapy services in psychogeriatrics

Time of day	Frequency	%
In the morning	8	(26.7%)
In the afternoon	1	(3.3%)
Morning and afternoon	7	(23.3%)
Afternoon and evening	1	(3.3%)
No preference	13	(43.3%)
n = 30		

Questions asked about music therapy practice with psychogeriatric patients were divided into two sections: receptive and active music therapy. For both receptive and active music therapy it was asked if the therapist preferred an individual or group approach. Most of the music therapists indicated that they worked equally often with groups as with individual therapy. Three music therapists indicated that they worked either solely with groups or solely with individual patients. When working in groups, on average the group consists of six clients (range two to fifteen clients). Both within individual therapy and during group therapy, a combination is preferred of receptive and active music therapy (Table 6.5). Most often a session starts with music listening that changes later in the session to an active form of music therapy.

Table 6.5 The use of receptive and active music therapy in individual and group therapy with psychogeriatric residents

	Individual therapy	Group therapy
I use mostly receptive music therapy	1 (3.6%)	1 (3.6%)
I use mostly active music therapy	1 (3.6%)	5 (17.9%)
Both receptive and active music therapy	26 (92.9%)	22 (78.6%)
n = 28		

This corresponds with the study of Drieschner and Pioch (1998) in which it was concluded that active and receptive music therapy was equally often used with group or individual therapy. In comparison to other clinical populations, receptive music therapy was used far more often with elderly people.

Receptive music therapy with psychogeriatric patients

In the literature, the process of a client listening to music is often described as 'passive music therapy'. In the Netherlands, the preferred term is 'receptive music therapy' as music listening involves active processes on part of the listener. Receptive music not only includes the residents listening to music played on audio equipment but also implies that the residents listen to the music the music therapist plays or sings. Most music therapists (25 therapists or 89.3%) use both forms of receptive music therapy. On average, a receptive music therapy session takes 38 minutes (minimum 15 minutes – maximum 90 minutes). It is often stated in the literature that preferably familiar music is chosen for the residents. In this survey it was asked which musical repertoire is used during receptive music therapy with psychogeriatric residents.

The option most often selected was classical music whereas New Age music was the least preferred. Other types of music that were reported included one's own musical repertoire, improvised music, music from the time when the resident was a child and religious music.

Table 6.6 Musical repertoire used in receptive music therapy	
Musical repertoire	Frequency
I do not use existent musical repertoire	5 (17.9%)
Music based on musical preferences of the patient	25 (89.3%)
Music from the time when the patient was a young adult	24 (85.7%)
Classical music	28 (100.0%)
Folk music	20 (71.4%)
Popular music	18 (64.35%)
New Age music	13 (46.4%)
Nature sounds	15 (53.6%)
n = 28	

In the music psychology literature, specific instruments are seen as being more suitable than others to convey a particular emotion. Gabrielson and Juslin (1996) instructed nine professional musicians to sing or play – on violin, flute or electrical guitar – particular emotional expressions such as happiness, sadness and anger as well as without expression. In general, the listener easily understood which emotional expression was played or sung. The researchers concluded that the effect is influenced by the type of musical instrument or whether one sings an emotional expression. Behrens and Green (1993) stated in their research that the violin and singing were more suitable to express sadness.

If there is such an effect of instruments during music therapy, it is as yet unstated, although it can be assumed that there is a clear relation between the type of music played and the feelings it induces in the client. Table 6.7 lists which instruments are present in both receptive and active approaches. Singing is also included.

Table 6.7 Instruments present in receptive and active music therapy		
Type of instrument	Frequency of use in receptive music therapy	Frequency of use in active music therapy
Keyboard instruments: piano, accordion, keyboard, organ	32	29
String instruments: guitar, violin, zither, lute, psaltery, chrotta	27	19
Singing	19	20
Percussion instruments: claves, vibraphone, chimes, xylophone, timpani, drums, gongs, rattles	18	80
Wind instruments: flute, mouth organ	11	4
	n = 27	n = 30

Next an open-ended question was asked according to which goals music therapists work within receptive music therapy, in both individual and group therapy (Table 6.8). On average three goals were reported for both individual and group therapy.

Active music therapy with geriatric residents

During active music therapy the residents are actively involved in the process of music-making in various musical activities. Overall twenty-six (92.9%) therapists reported that they used a combination of active and receptive music therapy in individual therapy and twenty-two (78.6%) when conducting group therapy. The use of mostly active music therapy was reported by one music therapist who solely worked with individual therapy. Five music therapists reported a mostly active music therapy approach when they worked with groups. The average time spent in active music therapy is similar

Table 6.8 Goals in receptive individual and group music therapy with psychogeriatric residents

Receptive individual music therapy	Frequency	Receptive group music therapy	Frequency
Relaxation	19	Sense of group and social contact	11
Stimulating communication and contact	15	Reminiscence: adjusting to personal memories and experiences	10
Reminiscence: adjusting to personal memories and experiences	8	Relaxation	8
Activation	6	Pleasure and experience of positive feelings	5
Acceptance and grief	6	Establishing contact and communication	5
Stimulating expression of feelings	5	Stimulating expression of feelings	4
Influencing mood states	5	Working on self-esteem and autonomy	3
n = 27		n = 25	

to receptive music therapy. On average an active music therapy session takes 40 minutes (minimum 20 minutes – maximum 60 minutes).

Whereas in receptive music therapy, an existing musical repertoire is used, active music therapy prefers predominantly musical improvisation. Fifteen music therapists (48.4%) indicated that they do not use existent musical repertoire during active music therapy, where the most reported option was the use of music based on the musical preferences of the residents. The least preferred musical repertoire within active music therapy was New Age music and nature sounds (see Table 6.9).

While goals in receptive individual music therapy are primarily related to relaxation, in individual active music therapy the most reported goals are strengthening self-esteem and stimulating expression. Within active group

Table 6.9 Musical repertoire used in active music therapy	
Musical repertoire	Frequency
I do not use existent musical repertoire	15 (48.4%)
Music based on musical preferences of the patient	28 (90.3%)
Music from the time when the patient was a young adult	21 (67.7%)
Classical music	18 (58.1%)
Folk music	21 (67.7%)
Popular music	16 (51.6%)
New Age music	6 (19.4%)
Nature sounds	7 (22.6%)
n = 31	

therapy the focus is on improving social contact and letting the clients experience that they belong to a group. The most frequent reported goals are listed in Table 6.10. On average four goals were reported, both for individual and group therapy.

While in receptive music therapy melodic instruments were most frequently mentioned, in active music therapy percussion and rhythm instruments are preferred (see Table 6.7). As the level of communication in music therapy is predominantly non-verbal, music therapy is one of the few approaches in which residents of varying levels of functioning can participate without the higher functioning residents dominating. One resident can still sing along with the well-known songs from the past, whereas another can move along to the beat of the music or play a small rhythm instrument, such as claves.

While often stated that music therapy has a beneficial effect with demented elderly people, relatively unknown is why music has such a strong effect. Psychogeriatric residents still continue to sing despite aphasia. While language deterioration is a feature of cognitive deficit, musical abilities appear to be preserved (Aldridge 1996). It has been stated by various researchers that language processing is dominant in one hemisphere and

Table 6.10 Goals in active individual and group music therapy with psychogeriatric residents

Receptive individual music therapy	Frequency	Receptive group music therapy	Frequency
Strengthening sense of self-esteem and self-confidence	15	Establishing a sense of belonging to a group, improving social contact and social awareness	17
Stimulating expression	14	Improving communication and sparing current social abilities	15
Establishing contact	13	Improving sense of self-esteem and autonomy	10
Regulating fear, aggression and anxiety	10	Expression of emotion and sharing of emotion	9
Providing pleasure and comfort	5	Providing pleasure and comfort	6
Influencing affect and reinforcing positive emotions	5	Relaxation	5
Relaxation	4	Acceptance of losses and grief	4
Acceptance of losses and grief	3	Improving concentration	4

music production involves an understanding of the interaction of both hemispheres (Altenmüller 1986; Brust 1980; Gates and Bradshaw 1977), which could explain why aphasic patients can still sing and that musical skills remain preserved.

It can be assumed, as it is seen with early infant caretaker interactions, that melodic intonations are an essential component in communication with demented elderly people. Possibly, the fundamentals of language are musical, and prior to lexical functions in language development (Aldridge 1996). Others have referred to the Progressively Lowered Stress Threshold Model (Hall and Buckwalter 1987) in the context of dementia. Following this model, the threshold for experiencing stress lowers as a result of declining cognitive and social skills. According to Hall and Buckwalter (1987), maximum functional levels can be achieved not by challenging to regain lost functions but by compensating for those losses. As musical abilities are longer preserved the losses can be compensated. Following this model the music activities should fit the abilities of the individual to obtain optimal participation.

It was questioned how music therapists themselves explain the effect of music with psychogeriatric residents. The most often mentioned option was that music directly appeals to feelings and emotions. It was also frequently mentioned that music is communication and music, therefore, has such a strong effect, especially with elderly people with whom verbal communication is no longer possible. Music is also considered as a strong cue to evoke memories and pleasant associations.

Music therapy and Alzheimer's disease patients

The last section of the questionnaire involved music therapy practice with a particular group: Alzheimer's disease patients. In the literature the effect of music therapy with Alzheimer's disease patients has often been the focus of research. Social behaviour has been found to increase through the use of music (Pollack and Namazi 1992). Negative behaviours such as wandering decrease (Groene 1993) and even cognitive skills have been found to improve (Prickett and Moore 1991). Music therapists indicated that they had an average of five years' experience in working with this client group.

Most music therapists agreed with the statements that music therapy decreases physical aggressive behaviour and that music therapy improves social skills. The statement they most often disagreed with was that music therapy can improve memory skills in Alzheimer's patients.

In an open-ended question music therapists were asked which goals they adhere to in their work with Alzheimer's disease patients (see Table 6.11). The goal most frequently mentioned was establishing contact and improving social skills. There were no typical goals that were especially mentioned for working with Alzheimer's disease patients in comparison with psychogeriatrics in general.

Table 6.11 Goals in working with Alzheimer's disease patients

Goals	Frequency
Establishing contact and improving social skills	17
Relaxation	13
Self-esteem, strengthening self-confidence	11
Providing a sense of safety and trust	6
Grief and acceptance of lost abilities	5
n = 27	

Dementia is typically characterized by a progressive decline in functions which is often described in three sequential stages: the early, middle and last stage of dementia. Most of the questions involving specific music therapy techniques related to Alzheimer's disease patients were related to three disease phases. A description of these stages was provided based on Reisberg *et al.* (1982). The first stage of the disease is characterized by a decrease in memory functions, disorientation and the first changes in personality. The middle stage of the disease is often longer in duration and is described as the stage in which memory functions further decrease associated with an increase in major psychiatric disorders such as hallucinations and psychoses and an increase in behavioural disorders such as verbal and physical aggression. The last stage of the disease is characterized by a continuing decrease in overall functioning: the inability to speak, incontinence, family members are no longer recognized, and the loss of psychomotor skills. The patient becomes bedridden and will eventually die.

Music therapists were asked if they worked with mostly individual or group therapy during each of these three phases (see Table 6.12). In the first phase, therapists prefer group therapy or indicated a preference for both group and individual therapy. As can be seen from this table there is a transition from the choice of group therapy to individual therapy, depending on the level of functioning of the patients. Music therapists opted more frequently for individual therapy for residents in the last phase of dementia. Where a group approach is used, on average the group consists of five to seven participants.

That the choice of active versus receptive music therapy depended on the level of functioning of the residents was also questioned (see Table 6.13). A combination of receptive and active music therapy is mostly used for residents in the first and middle stage of dementia, whereas in the third stage music therapists prefer receptive music therapy, when functioning levels of the residents are minimal. On average the active music therapy sessions take about 42 minutes whereas receptive music therapy sessions take about 39 minutes.

	Table 6.12 Preference for individual and group therapy related to disease progression		
	First stage	Second stage	Third stage
Individual therapy	1	3	15
Group therapy	10	3	0
Both	12	20	10
	n = 23	n = 26	n = 25

	Table 6.13 Preference for receptive or active music therapy related to disease progression		
	First stage	Second stage	Third stage
Active music therapy	5	6	0
Receptive music therapy	1	1	19
Both	17	19	6
	n = 23	n = 26	n = 25

Discussion

This survey revealed that there is currently a well-qualified group of music therapists working in psychogeriatric care in the Netherlands. Most music therapists work eclectically and refer to their colleagues for further information on recent developments in music therapy. Active and receptive music therapy is equally applied in practice and depends on the level of functioning of the client. When the level of functioning of the client decreases, more therapists opt for an individualistic approach and use receptive approaches.

This study is limited in the scope of work-related aspects that it addresses. Further questions that can be asked are: How does a music therapist decide which techniques to use with a specific client population? How do ways of working differ between different client populations and with what effect? These questions are essential to learn more of the effect of music therapy and to argue for referral to music therapy. More descriptive in-depth research of specific areas of music therapy practice would be welcome.

Engelman (1995) describes that there are currently more psychiatric institutions in Germany with a music therapist than without. Unfortunately, this is still not the case for psychogeriatric care in the Netherlands. An important reason is that music activities in psychogeriatrics are often conducted by 'occupational therapists'. In most cases, Dutch nursing homes do know about the beneficial effects of music but they often do not know about the beneficial effects of music therapy. A lack of information about music therapy contributes to this situation as little is published on the topic of music therapy in the general health-care journals.

In reference to the use of receptive versus active music therapy, it should be underlined that receptive music therapy is highly undervalued in the Netherlands. During training and in the literature, the emphasis is often on active musical improvisation. With this client population, receptive music therapy is very useful. Hand co-ordination often fails when the elderly residents become increasingly frail, and receptive music techniques are the only option to let the residents benefit from music's potential.

Acknowledgements

This study is supported by grants from the Dutch Alzheimer Foundation (Alzheimer Nederland), Triodos Foundation, Fund Music Therapy of Buma Stemra and the Rens Holle Foundation.

CHAPTER 7

Improvisation as an Assessment of Potential in Early Alzheimer's Disease

Gudrun Aldridge

After completing two major concertos for the piano, the composer Maurice Ravel, at the age of 56, began to complain of increased fatigue and lassitude. Following a traffic accident his condition deteriorated progressively (Henson 1988). He lost the ability to remember names, to speak spontaneously and to write (Dalessio 1984). Although he could understand speech, he was no longer capable of the co-ordination required to lead a major orchestra. While his mind, he reports, was full of musical ideas, he could not set them down (Dalessio 1984). Eventually his intellectual functions and speech deteriorated until he could no longer recognize his own music. We would speculate now that he had been suffering from Alzheimer's disease.

In this chapter, the value of music for the sufferers of Alzheimer's disease will be discussed. In particular, I shall present improvisation as an assessment of potential in early Alzheimer's disease and illustrate it with an analysis of musical examples. As this material was gathered within the context of therapy in a hospital clinic, I shall further demonstrate how the assessment serves as a basis for developing criteria from which I identify therapeutic goals and develop therapeutic strategies.

Music as therapy

There are two principal ways of doing music therapy: 'active music therapy', which requires that the patient or a group of patients play musical instruments, or sing, with the therapist, and 'passive music therapy', whereby the patient or a group of patients listen to the therapist, who plays live or recorded music to them. Of course, the act of listening itself is an activity and is rarely passive.

In active music therapy, the music is often improvised to suit the individual patient. In passive music therapy, the music is often chosen to suit particular patients. Within each of these two main approaches, there are varying schools throughout the western world, some based on the work of particular teachers, some more eclectic and based on psychotherapeutic approaches, others claiming to be a 'music-medicine'. Music therapy has been reviewed in the medical and nursing press and the principal emphasis is on the soothing ability of music and the necessity of music as an antidote to an overly technological medical approach. Most of these articles are concerned with passive music therapy and the playing of pre-recorded music to patients emphasizing the necessity of healthy pleasures like music, fragrance and beautiful sights for the reduction of stress and the enhancement of well-being and the overall expectation is that the recreational, emotional and physical health of the patient is improved (Aldridge 1993b, 1996).

However, after the Second World War music therapy was intensively developed in American hospitals (Schullian and Schoen 1948). Since then some hospitals, particularly in mainland Europe, have incorporated music therapy carrying on a tradition of European hospital-based research and practice (Aldridge 1990; Aldridge, Brandt and Wohler 1989). In recent years there has been a move to develop an academic tradition of research that attempts to begin a clinical dialogue with other practitioners through research practice (Aldridge 1989, 1991a, 1991b, 1993a, 1996; Aldridge, Gustorff and Hannich 1990).

Music, cognition and language

As in Ravel's demise, the responsiveness of patients with Alzheimer's disease to music is a remarkable phenomenon (Swartz *et al.* 1989). While language deterioration is a feature of cognitive deficit, musical abilities appear to be preserved. This may be because the fundamentals of language are musical, and prior to semantic and lexical functions in language development.

Although language processing may be dominant in one hemisphere of the brain, music production involves an understanding of the interaction of both cerebral hemispheres (Altenmüller 1986; Brust 1980; Gates and Bradshaw 1977). In attempting to understand the perception of music there have been a number of investigations into the hemispheric strategies involved. Much of the literature considering musical perception concentrates on the significance of hemispheric dominance. Gates and Bradshaw (1977) conclude that cerebral hemispheres are concerned with music perception and that no laterality differences are apparent. Other authors (Wagner and Hannon 1981) suggest that two processing functions develop with training where left and right hemispheres are simultaneously involved, and that musical stimuli are capable of eliciting both right and left ear superiority (Kellar and Bever 1980). Similarly, when people listen to and perform music they utilize differing hemispheric processing strategies.

Evidence of the global strategy of music processing in the brain is found in the clinical literature. In two cases of aphasia (Morgan and Tilluckdharry 1982) singing was seen as a welcome release from the helplessness of being a patient. The author hypothesized that singing was a means to communicate thoughts externally. Although the 'newer aspect' of speech was lost, the older function of music was retained possibly because music is a function distributed over both hemispheres. Berman (1981) suggests that recovery from aphasia is not a matter of new learning by the non-dominant hemisphere but a taking over of responsibility for language by that hemisphere. The non-dominant hemisphere may be a reserve of functions in case of regional failure.

Little is known about the loss of musical and language abilities in cases of global cortical damage, although the quality of response to music in the final stages of dementia is worth noting (Norberg et al. 1986). Any discussion is necessarily limited to hypothesizing as there are no established baselines for musical performance in the adult population (Swartz et al. 1989).

Aphasia, which is a feature of cognitive deterioration, is a complicated phenomenon. While syntactical functions may remain longer, it is the lexical and semantic functions of naming and reference, which begin to fail in the early stages. Phrasing and grammatical structures remain giving an impression of normal speech, yet content becomes increasingly incoherent. These progressive failings appear to be located within the context of semantic and episodic memory loss illustrated by the inability to remember a simple story when tested (Bayles et al. 1989).

Musicality and singing are rarely tested as features of cognitive deterioration, yet preservation of these abilities in aphasics has been linked to eventual recovery (Jacome 1984; Morgan and Tilluckdharry 1982) and could be significant indicators of hierarchical changes in cognitive functioning. Jacome (1984) found that a musically naïve patient with transcortical mixed aphasia exhibited repetitive, spontaneous whistling and whistling in response to questions. The patient often spontaneously sang without error in pitch, melody, rhythm and lyrics, and spent long periods of time listening to music. In a study by Moore, Staum and Brotons (1992) patients remembered the words of songs they had sung during therapy sessions better than spoken material. The percentage of recall was better for older than for newer songs. Beatty *et al.* (1988) describe a woman who had severe impairments in terms of aphasia, memory dysfunction and apraxia yet was able to sight read an unfamiliar song and perform on the xylophone which to her was an unconventional instrument. Like Ravel (Dalessio 1984) and an elderly musician who could play from memory but no longer recalled the name of the composer, she no longer recalled the title of the music she was playing.

Swartz *et al.* (1989) propose a series of perceptual levels at which musical disorders take place:

1.   the acoustico-psychological level, which includes changes in intensity, pitch and timbre

2.   the discriminatory level, which includes the discrimination of intervals and chords

3.   the categorical level, which includes the categorical identification of rhythmic patterns and intervals

4.   the configurable level, which includes melody perception, the recognition of motifs and themes, tonal changes, identification of instruments and rhythmic discrimination

5.   the level where musical form is recognized, including complex perceptual and executive functions of harmonic, melodic and rhythmical transformations.

In Alzheimer's patients it would be expected that while levels (1), (2) and (3) remain unaffected, the complexities of levels (4) and (5), when requiring no naming, may be preserved but are susceptible to deterioration.

It is perhaps important to point out that these disorders are not themselves musical, they are disorders of audition. Only when disorders of musical production take place can we begin to suggest that a musical disorder is present. Improvised musical playing is in an unique position to demonstrate this hypothetical link between perception and production.

Rhythm is the key to the integrative process underlying both musical perception and physiological coherence. When considering communication, rhythm is also fundamental to the organization and co-ordination of internal processes, and externally between. Rhythm offers a frame of reference for perception (Povel 1984).

Rhythm too plays a role in the perception of melody. The perceptions of speech and music are formidable tasks of pattern perception. The listener has to extract meaning from lengthy sequences of rapidly changing elements. Temporal predictability is important for tracking melody lines (Aldridge 1993a). Kidd, Boltz and Jones (1984) also refer to melody as having a structure in time and that a regular rhythm facilitates the detection of a musical interval and its subsequent integration into a cognitive representation of the serial structure of the musical pattern. Adults identify familiar melodies on the basis of relational information about intervals between tones rather than the absolute information of particular tones. In the recognition of unfamiliar melodies, less precise information is gathered about the tone itself. The primary concern is with successive frequency changes or melodic contour. The rhythmical context prepares the listener in advance for the onset of certain musical intervals and therefore a structure from which to discern, or predict, change. One may not be aware of certain changes and become either out of tune or out of time; such a loss of rhythmical structure, which appears outwardly as confusion, may be a hidden factor in the understanding of Alzheimer's disease.

What is important in these descriptions of musical perception is the emphasis on context where there are different levels of attention occurring simultaneously against a background temporal structure. Musical improvisation with a therapist, which emphasizes attention to the environment utilizing changes in tempo and volition, without regard for lexical content, may be an ideal medium for treatment initiatives with Alzheimer's patients. The playing of simple rhythmic patterns and melodic phrases by the therapist, and the expectation that the patient will copy those patterns or phrases, is similar to the element of 'registration' in the mental state examination (Aldridge 1996).

While improvised musical playing is a useful tool for the assessment of musical abilities, it is as in this case also used within a therapeutic context. In this way assessment and therapy are interlinked – assessment providing the criteria from which to identify therapeutic goals and develop therapeutic strategies.

Music therapy and elderly people

Much of the published work concerning music therapy with elderly people is concerned with group activity (Bryant 1991; Christie 1992; Olderog-Millard and Smith 1989) and is generally used to expand socialization and communication skills, with the intention of reducing problems of social isolation and withdrawal, to encourage participants to interact purposefully with others, assist in expressing and communicating feelings and ideas, and to stimulate cognitive processes, thereby sharpening problem-solving skills. Additional goals also focus on sensory and muscular stimulation and gross and fine motor skill development (Segal 1990).

As we have seen in Chapter 4, Clair has worked extensively with elderly people and found music therapy a valuable tool for working in groups to promote communicating, watching others, singing, interacting with an instrument, and sitting. Wandering, confusion and agitation are linked problems common to elderly patients living in hostels or special accommodation for Alzheimer's patients. A music therapist (Fitzgerald-Cloutier 1993) has tested singing with an 81-year-old woman to see if it helped her to remain seated. After 20 singing sessions, the therapist read to the woman to compare the degree of attentiveness. While music therapy and reading sessions redirected the woman from wandering, the total time she sat for the music therapy sessions was double that of the reading sessions (214.3 minutes versus 99.1 minutes) and the time spent seated in the music therapy was more consistent than the sporadic episodes when she was being read to. When agitation occurs in such elderly women, then individualized music therapy appears to have a significantly calming effect (Gerdner and Swanson 1993). In terms of reducing repetitive behaviour, musical activity also reduces disruptive vocalizations (Casby and Holm 1994).

The above conclusions are supported by Groene (1993): 30 residents (aged 60–91 years) in a special Alzheimer's unit, who exhibited wandering behaviour, were randomly assigned to either mostly music attention or mostly reading attention groups where they received one-to-one attention. Those receiving music therapy remained seated longer than those did in the reading sessions.

One of the central problems of elderly people is the loss of independence and self-esteem. Palmer (1977, 1983, 1989) describes a programme of music therapy at a geriatric home designed to rebuild self-concept. For the 380 residents, ranging from those who were totally functional to those who needed total care, a programme was adapted to the capacities and needs of individual patients. Marching and dancing increased the ability of some patients to walk well; and for the non-ambulatory, kicking and stamping to music improved circulation and increased tolerance and strength. Sing-along sessions were used to encourage memory recall and promoted social interaction and appropriate social behaviour (Palmer 1983, 1989). It was such social behaviour that Pollack and Namazi (1992) report as being accessible to improvement through group music therapy activities. It is the participative element, that appears to be valuable for communication, and the intention to participate that is at the core of the music therapy activity, which we shall see in the following section.

Music therapy has also been used to focus on memory recall for songs and the spoken word (Prickett and Moore 1991). In ten elderly patients, whose diagnosis was probably Alzheimer's disease, words to songs were recalled dramatically better than spoken words or spoken information. Although long-familiar songs were recalled with greater accuracy than a newly presented song, most patients attempted to sing, hum or keep time while the therapist sang. However, it could be that other factors such as tempo, length of seconds per word, and total number of words that might be more closely associated with lyric recall than the relative familiarity of the song selection.

In a further study of the effects of three treatment approaches, musically cued reminiscence, verbally cued reminiscence, and music alone, on the cognitive functioning of twelve female nursing home residents with Alzheimer's disease, changes in cognitive functioning were assessed by the differences between pre- and post-session treatment scores on the Mini-Mental State Examination. Comparisons were made for total scores and sub-scores for orientation, attention and language. Musically cued and verbally cued reminiscence significantly increased language subsection scores and musical activity alone significantly increased total scores (G. Smith 1986).

Prinsley (1986) recommends music therapy for geriatric care as it reduces the individual prescription of tranquillizing medication, reduces the use of hypnotics on the hospital ward and helps overall rehabilitation. He recommends that music therapy be based on treatment objectives; the social goals of interaction co-operation; psychological goals of mood improvement and self-expression; intellectual goals of the stimulation of speech and organization of mental processes; and the physical goals of sensory stimulation and motor integration. Such goals as stimulation of the individual, promoting involvement in social activity, identifying specific individualized behavioural targets, and emphasizing the maintenance of specific memory functions is repeated throughout the music therapy literature (Prange 1990; S. Smith 1990; Summer 1981). Similarly, D. Smith (1990) recommends behavioural interventions targeted at the more common behavioural problems (e.g. disorientation, age-related changes in social activity, sleep disturbances) of institutionalized elderly persons. In a study of music therapy in two nursing homes, life satisfaction and self-esteem were significantly improved in the home where the residents participated in the musical activities (VanderArk, Newman and Bell 1983) in comparison with a matched control group that had no music therapy.

Music therapy with an Alzheimer's patient: a case study

In this case example I first want to outline my music therapeutic approach and then describe the music therapeutic events carried out with a female patient. The music therapy I describe here is based upon the improvisation of music between therapist and patient (Nordoff and Robbins 1977). The music therapist creates and improvises the music with the patient using a range of instruments. This work often begins with an exploratory session using rhythmic instruments; progressing to the use of rhythmic/melodic instruments such as the chime bars, glockenspiel or xylophone; developing into work with melodic instruments (including the piano) and the voice. In this way of working the emphasis is on a series of musical improvisations during each session, and music is the vehicle for the therapy. Musical assessment and therapy are interlinked, providing the criteria from which to identify therapeutic goals. Each session is audio tape-recorded, with the consent of the patient, and later analysed and indexed as to musical content. No musical training is required of the patient.

Music therapy is used here as one modality of a comprehensive treatment package. A 55-year-old female patient was referred initially to the hospital when she, and her family, became aware of her deteriorating condition. Her sister had died with Alzheimer's disease, and the family were concerned that she too was repeating her sister's demise as her memory became increasingly disturbed. At home she was experiencing difficulties in finding items of clothing and other things necessary for everyday life. She could not go shopping and cook for herself any more and was unable to write her own name. While wanting to speak, she experienced difficulty in finding words. Her vocabulary was reduced to short phrases. She also appeared to be depressed, and in the light of her sister's death, and her own knowledge regarding her current predicament, it seemed reasonable to make this assumption. It is worth mentioning that at the age of 40 she had been actively making music at home. She began playing the piano for family, friends and acquaintances, although without any formal studies. Her musical activity had disappeared in her late forties. Given this earlier, and not too distant, musical interest, music therapy appeared to have potential as an intervention adjuvant to medical treatment.

Beginning therapy

The patient was unable to find her way on public transport and was brought to the hospital by her son for ten weekly sessions. Each session lasted for about 40 minutes.

The neuropsychiatrist believed that music therapy was indicated. She further included anthroposophical treatment with the goal of delaying the progress of the dementia in its overall course.

My questions regarding the improvisations were as follows:

- Does this disease make its appearance in the musical playing of the patient?

- Is it possible to include the musicality (i.e. the musical abilities) of the patient into the therapeutic process?

- What possibilities can music therapy offer as complementary to medical and other therapeutic interventions?

- Is it possible to make a comparison between medical and music therapeutic components of assessment?

Rhythmic playing

In all ten sessions the patient demonstrated her ability to play, without my influence, a singular ordered rhythmic pattern in 4/4 time using two sticks on a single drum. This rhythmical pattern appeared in various forms and can be portrayed as in Figure 7.1.

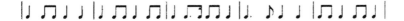

Figure 7.1 A singular ordered rhythmic pattern

A feature of her rhythmical playing was that in nearly all sessions, during the progress of an improvisation, the patient would let control of the rhythmic pattern slip such that it became progressively imprecise, losing both its form and liveliness. The initial impulse of her rhythmical playing, which was clear and precise, gradually deteriorated as she lost concentration and ability to persevere with the task in hand. However, when I offered an overall musical structure during the course of the improvisation by playing her a known piece of music then the patient could regain her precision of rhythm.

This fact will be demonstrated in the musical example (Figure 7.2).

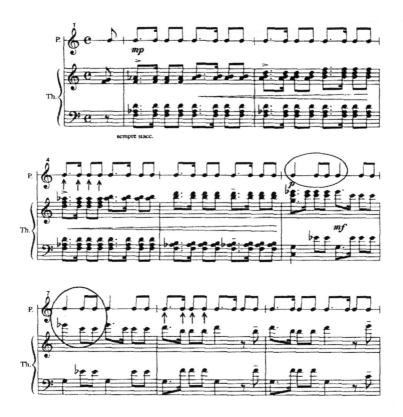

Figure 7.2 Losing the structure of the rhythm

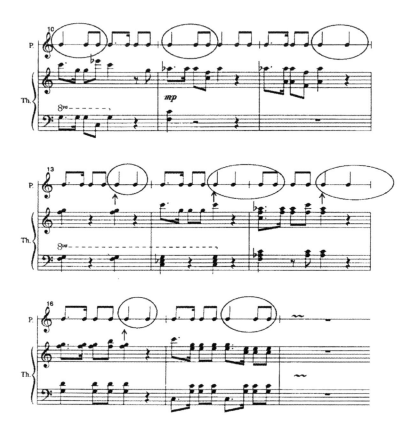

Figure 7.2 (continued...) Losing the structure of the rhythm

Figure 7.2 shows the score of the patient's and therapist's voices. In order to involve the patient in an active rhythmical playing I introduced a pattern, characterized by an upbeat and a dotted note (Example 7a).

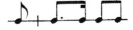

Example 7a

We can see in the voice of the therapist (bars 1–6) that the gradual tension-building by pitch and dynamic in diminished harmonic progression in combination with a precise articulation helped the patient to hold the pattern until the peak was reached (bar 6). At the turn of the peak (bar 6) the patient lost the grip of the dotted pattern. It is due to her inherent musicality that this slippage turned into an even form of rhythm without interruption (Example 7b).

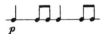

Example 7b

This process of letting an initial pattern slip is recognizable in the following bars (7–17) of the patient's score (see marked notes). When the patient was directly supported by me with the same pattern she could sometimes regain the initial dotted note (bars 8, 12). However, when I gave room for her voice and drew back from voice-volume and continuing playing, the patient reduced her musical activity as is shown in her rhythmical extension (bars 12, 13–16).

Although she lost access to one single element, like rhythmical detail, she was still in contact with her inner musicality, being related to the basic order of tempo and beat.

The patient reacted to changes in time and musical forms and incorporated them within her playing. Significantly she responded to changes of form from 4/4 to 3/4, often remarking 'now it is a waltz' or 'now it becomes quieter'.

The notation in Figure 7.3 reveals her awareness to changes in music and her way of response. A change of time occurs from 4/4 (bar 6) to 3/4 (bar 7). While the patient was actively participating on the drum to the basic movement of 4/4 time, emphasizing the march-like character of the music (bars 1–5) she noticed a change in the music and made a comment on this: 'now it becomes quieter' (bar 4). It is interesting to see that she realized a change in the music but could not seize and name it precisely. In fact the music played by me changed to the repetition of a melodic motif, taken from the preceding phrase (see Figure 7.3, bars 1–2) Accompanied by rests (bars

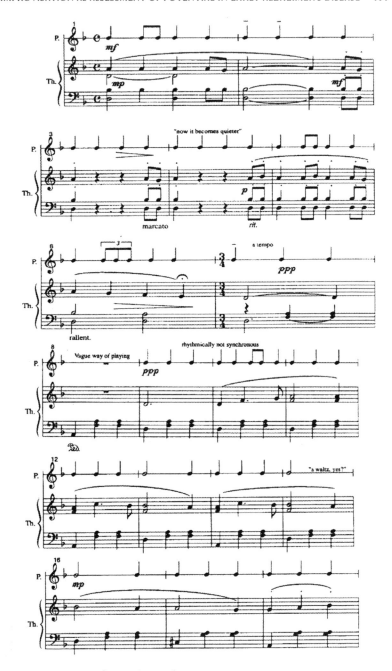

Figure 7.3 Her way of responding to changes in music

3–4), this motif was brought out by a change in articulation and stronger dynamic (see Example 7c).

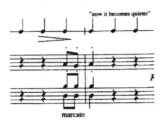

Example 7c

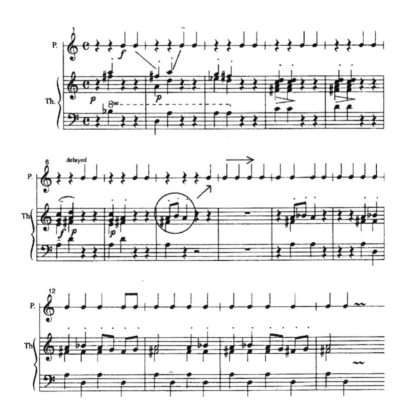

Figure 7.4 Difficulty in realizing changes in pattern

It became obvious that it was the interruption of the flow of music by rests that caused the patient's comment 'now it becomes quieter'. This would support the perceptual levels (see levels 4 and 5) proposed by Swartz *et al.* (1989), mentioned earlier, at which musical disorders take place. Here we can discern the lack of identifying and recognizing a melodic motif out of a context and the lack of perceptual and executive transfer.

Another feature points to the fact that in the moment the patient started to speak, her attention was withdrawn from her current activity so that her playing became weaker in expression (bar 3).

The actual change of time was introduced by ritardando (bar 6) and a descending melodic line, supported by my voice. Looking at the patient's score we can discern that the patient temporarily fell out of time, losing the rhythmical structure. But, after having experienced the new time signature in playing it in a more stable way (bars 11–14), she was able to identify the change and remark on it with 'a waltz, yes?' (bar 15).

Figure 7.4 demonstrates the patient's difficulty to perceive and convert a change in pattern. This change in pattern occurred within the form of a dialogue.

The patient had no difficulty in keeping possession of her playing within the established exchange of a simple two-beat pattern (bars 1–7) (see also Example 7d).

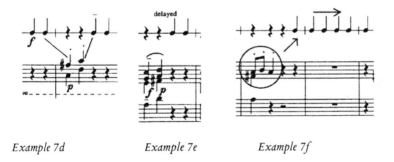

Example 7d   *Example 7e*   *Example 7f*

She was entirely taken up by this pattern but could not respond to other musical features like dynamic and articulation. In bar 6 we can recognize her delayed answer caused by the introduction of dynamic contrast: forte/piano (see Example 7e). When the actual change of pattern occurred (bar 8) the patient again responded with delay, giving up her complementary participation that led her to continuous playing (Example 7f).

These rhythmical improvisations, using different drums and cymbals, were played in later sessions on two instruments together. On one instrument the patient showed no difficulty in co-ordinating parallel or alternate-handed playing on a single instrument. She could maintain her rhythmical activity when played within a fluent tempo of about 120 beats per minute and in a narrow dynamic range (mp–mf). However, the introduction of two instruments brought a major difficulty for the patient, who stood disoriented before the instruments, unable to integrate them both in her playing. It was only with instruction and direction from me that she was able to co-ordinate right–left playing on two instruments.

Melodic playing

Melodic playing was a critical point in therapy because in trying to play a melody on chime bars or metallophone the patient became aware of her deterioration. The patient knew several folksongs from earlier times and was able to sing them along with me. After only a few notes played by me on the piano, she could associate them with a well-known tune. However, when she tried to play a complete melody on the piano or other instruments then it proved impossible. Although beginning spontaneously and fluently, she had difficulty in completing a known melody. When I played short initial motifs of familiar melodies the patient needed a lot of concentration to focus on her implementation. She often tried to support herself by simultaneously singing, bringing the two different actions of playing and singing together. Failure caused her frustration and distress.

At the introduction of a new melodic motif, she would often seek a melody known to her, rather than face the insecurity of an unknown improvised melody.

Another difficulty was that instruments, like metallophone and xylophone, which were previously unknown to her, remained forever strange. When I sat opposite her and showed her which notes to play then she was able to follow my finger movements.

When presented with a limited range of tones she also had difficulty in playing them, which may have been compounded by visio-spatial difficulties. It is easier to strike the broad surface of a drum skin than the limited precise surface of adjacent chime bars.

Harmonic playing

A similar thing occurred when she played the piano and tried to accompany a melody. At the beginning of her very first session she followed her impulse to play spontaneously on the piano and tried to play 'Happy is the gypsy life'. She easily accompanied the first part of this song harmonically with thirds and triads. The second part proved to be more difficult as she failed to find the subdominant, whereupon she broke off from the playing and remarked 'that always catches me out'.

This pattern of spontaneously striking up a melody, and then breaking off when the harmony failed, was to be repeated whenever she tried other melodies. She showed a fine musical sensitivity for the appropriate harmony, which was not always at her disposal to be played.

When playing on the drum, her musical sensitivity in her reactions to the contrasting sound qualities of major and minor was reduced but overall she had a pronounced perception of the harmonic realm of music. Musical functioning demonstrates something that similar in tests of language functioning; production is impaired while perception remains.

Therapeutic changes

In rhythmical playing on drum and cymbal, I attempted to develop the patient's attention span through the use of short repeated musical patterns and changes in key, volume and tempo. I hoped through these musical changes to steer her to maintaining a stable musical form. This technique helped the patient to maintain a rhythmical pattern and brought her to the stage in which she could express herself stronger musically. I also searched for other ways to develop variety in rhythm by moving away from the repetitive pattern played by the patient.

A change in the patient's ability to improvise was shown when she recognized, and could repeat rhythmical patterns in a musical dialogue and was thereby brought into a musical context.

In Figure 7.5 we see that the patient and I were first joined up in the basic movement of 4/4 (bars 1–4). The patient followed the ritardando that indicated the end of the preceding march-like piece. The ritardando brought about a momentary change in tempo causing the patient to loosen her grip. Loosening her grip indicated that the patient's attention dropped momentarily but was present again as soon as she recognized a pattern played by me (bars 4–5). Her response to this was not in time but she was able to correct herself (see Example 7g).

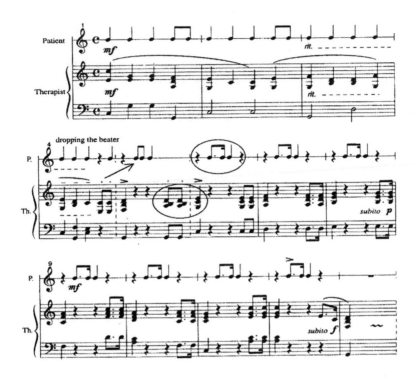

Figure 7.5 Recognizing a repeating rhythmical pattern

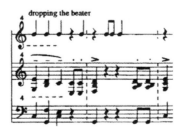

Example 7g

As soon as she regained contact to the basic time she was able to participate to a dialogue varying the pattern into a swinging expression appearing in form of dotted quaver (see Example 7h).

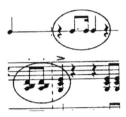

Example 7h

She was able to maintain the mutual exchange but would not additionally respond to dynamic variations (see Figure 7.5, bar 8: subito piano and bar 12 subito forte). On the one hand, the patient's concentration span concerning the maintenance of dialogic form was improved. On the other hand, she showed limitation to integrate further musical 'information'.

Taking 'dynamic' range as being one aspect of expression, it became obvious that the patient was not able to extend this possibility for herself. She displayed few changes in her dynamic playing and sometimes reacted to dynamic contrasts and transitions without awareness. The same thing could be seen in terms of her tempo range, which was set about 120 beats per minute and varied little.

In the end of the treatment phase of therapy, the patient was able to change her playing in this way such that she could express herself more strongly by bringing into line her thoughtful and affective playing. This ability to become rhythmically flexible, when incorporated into the form of a dialogue is a fundamental feature of encouraging communicational competence (Aldridge 1996).

Figure 7.6 illustrates her decision of changing her playing according to the character of the music and her musical satisfaction.

In Figure 7.6 we can see that the patient was able to integrate two instruments, drum and cymbal, within her musical playing. Her musical activity was related to time signature, rhythm and pitch. The gradual rise in pitch, played in octaves, encouraged her to emphasize the last beat of each

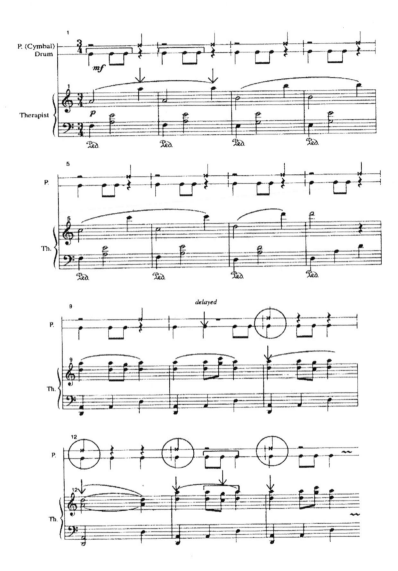

Figure 7.6 Changes of emphasis for fuller expression

bar. Corresponding to the top note of the octave (bar 1), she chose the contrasting sound of the cymbal (Example 7i).

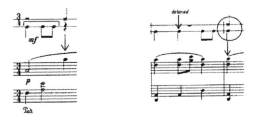

Example 7i   *Example 7j*

The patient stayed within her musical form until I introduced a new four-bar theme (bars 9–12) which I repeated and varied later. In bar 10 we can discover how the patient related to this musical change (Example 7j).

In perceiving the lively character of the new theme she slowed down, gave up her initial pattern and turned towards a new way of expression. According to the character of the music she changed the emphasis from the third to the first beat and intensified her decision by parallel hand movements (bar 11): see Example 7k.

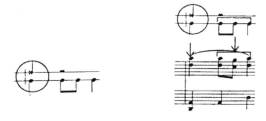

Example 7k   *Example 7l*

She continued in this way of organizing and shaping her accompaniment to the new music, regaining her initial pattern, which was part of the musical theme (see Example 7l).

The analysis of musical notation makes it possible to discover closely single elements of the patient's playing that appear when a musical change is taking place (see Figures 7.3, 7.4, 7.6). Although these events were demanding for the patient, they signified a concurrent motivating effect. She wanted to succeed, not to lose control and maintain coherence in what she could do.

As mentioned before, from the first session of therapy the patient made quite clear her intent to sit at the piano and play whatever melodies she chose and find the appropriate accompaniments. This wish, and the corresponding will-power to achieve this end, was shown in all the sessions. It was possible to use this impetus to play as a source for improvisation.

In the sixth session the patient improvised a rhythmical piece in 4/4 time, which I then transformed with a melodic phrase. At the end of the phrase the patient laughed with joy at the success of her playing and asked to play it again. The intent and expression with which she played could carry the original lapses and slips in the form of the rhythmical playing. While her overall intention to play was preserved, her attention to that playing, the concentration necessary for musical production and the perseverance required for completing a sequence of phrases progressively failed and was dependent on the overall musical structure offered by me. The music-therapeutic analysis of the examples reveal some features of the patient's therapeutic process and allow a detailed examination of what happens. It is in these very small changes that we can discern the musical therapeutic changes and the imperfections in perception.

Clinical changes

At the end of the treatment period, which also used homeopathic medicine, the patient was able to cook for herself and could find her own things about the house. The psychiatrist responsible for her therapeutic management reported an overall improvement in her interest in what was going on around her, and in particular, that she paid attention to visitors and maintained interest in conversations. The patient regained the ability to write her signature, although she could write only slowly. While wanting to speak, she still experienced difficulty in finding words.

It appears that music therapy had a beneficial effect on the quality of life for this patient. We cannot rule out that the therapy had an influence on an underlying depression and this may account for some of the therapeutic effect. While the patient came to the sessions with the intention of playing, her ability to take initiatives was impaired mirroring the state of her home life where she wanted to look after herself, yet was unable to take initiatives. I regarded this stimulus to take initiatives as an important feature of the music therapy. It appears that this impulse had a correlate in the way in which the patient began to take initiatives in her daily life.

Active music-making also promoted interaction thereby promoting initiatives in communication, which the patient also enjoyed, particularly when she accomplished playing a complete improvisation. The implications for the maintenance of memory by actively making music are significant as we have seen in Chapter 2. As Crystal *et al.* (1989) found in an 82-year-old musician with Alzheimer's disease, there was a preserved ability to play previously learned piano compositions from memory, although the man was unable to identify the composer or titles of each work. There was also a preserved ability to learn the new skill of mirror reading while being unable to recall or recognize new information.

A contra-indication for music therapy with such patients who are aware of their problems is that the awareness of further cognitive abilities as experienced in the playing may exacerbate any underlying depression and demotivate the patient to continue.

Conclusion

Alzheimer patients, despite aphasia and memory loss, continue to sing old songs and to dance to past tunes when given the chance. Indeed, fun and entertainment are all part of daily living for elderly people in special accommodation (Glassman 1983; Jonas 1991; Kartman 1990; B. Smith 1992). Quality of life expectations become paramount in any management strategy, and music therapy appears to play an important role in enhancing the ability to take part actively in daily life (Lipe 1991; Rosling and Kitchen 1992). However, the production of music and the improvisation of music appears to fail in the same way in which language fails.

If we are unsure as to the normal process of cognitive loss in ageing, we are even more in the dark as to the normal musical playing abilities of adults. The literature suggests that musical activities are preserved while other cognitive functions fail. Unfortunately no established guidelines as to the normal range of improvised music playing of adults is available.

Improvised music therapy appears to offer the opportunity to supplement mental state examinations in areas where those examinations are lacking. First, it is possible to ascertain the fluency of musical production. Second, intentionality, attention to, concentration on and perseverance with the task in hand are important features of producing musical improvisations and susceptible to being heard in the musical playing. Third, episodic memory can be tested in the ability to repeat short rhythmic and melodic phrases. The inability to build such phrases may be attributed to problems with memory or to a yet unknown factor. This unknown factor is possibly involved with the organization of time structures. If rhythmic structure is an overall context for musical production, and the ground structure for perception, it can be hypothesized that it is this overarching structure, which begins to fail in Alzheimer's patients. A loss of rhythmical context would explain why patients are able to produce and persevere with rhythmic and melodic playing when offered an overall structure by the therapist. Such a hypothesis would tie in with the musical hierarchy proposed by Swartz *et al.* (1989, p.154) and would suggest a global failing in cognition while localized lower abilities are retained. However, the hierarchy of musical perceptual levels proposed by Swartz *et al.* (1989) may need to be further subdivided into classifications of music reception and music production.

Music therapy appears to offer a sensitive assessment tool (see Tables 7.1 and 7.2). It tests those prosodic elements of speech production, which are not lexically dependent. Furthermore, it can be used to assess those areas of functioning, both receptive and productive, not covered adequately by other test instruments, that is fluency, perseverance in context, attention, concentration and intentionality. In addition it provides a form of therapy which may stimulate cognitive activities such that areas subject to progressive failure are maintained. Certainly the anecdotal evidence suggests that quality of life of Alzheimer's patients is significantly improved with music therapy (McCloskey 1985, 1990; Tyson 1989) accompanied by the overall social benefits of acceptance and sense of belonging gained by communicating with others (Morris 1986; Segal 1990).

In terms of research, single-case within-subject designs with Alzheimer's disease patients appear to be a feasible way forward to assess individual responses to musical interventions in the clinical realm. Such studies would depend upon careful clinical examinations, mental state examinations and musical assessments. Unfortunately most of the literature concerning cognition and musical perception is based upon audition and not musical production. Like other authors I suggest that the production of music, as is the production of language, be a complex global phenomenon as yet poorly understood. The understanding of musical production may well offer a clue to the ground structure of language and communication in general. It is research in this realm of perception, which is urgent not only for the under-

Table 7.1 Features of medical and musical elements of assessment

Medical elements of assessment	Musical elements of assessment
Continuing observation of mental and functional status	Continuing observation of mental and functional status
Testing of verbal skills, including element of speech fluency	Testing of musical skills: rhythm, melody, harmony, dynamic, phrasing, articulation
Cortical disorder testing: visio-spatial skills and ability to perform complex motor tasks (including grip and right–left co-ordination)	Cortical disorder testing: visio-spatial skills and ability to perform complex motor tasks (including grip and right–left co-ordination)
Testing for progressive memory disintegration	Testing for progressive memory disintegration
Motivation to complete tests, to achieve set goals and persevere in set tasks	Motivation to sustain playing improvised music, to achieve musical goals and persevere in maintaining musical form
'Intention' difficult to assess, but considered important	'Intention' a feature of improvised musical playing
Concentration and attention span	Concentration on the improvised playing and attention to the instruments
Flexibility in task switching	Flexibilty in musical (including instrumental) changes
Mini-Mental State Score influenced by educational status	Ability to play improvised music influenced by previous musical training
Insensitive to small changes	Sensitive to small changes
Ability to interpret surroundings	Ability to interpret musical context and assessment of communication in the therapeutic relationship

standing of Alzheimer's patients but also in the general context of cognitive deficit and brain behaviour. It may be as Berman (1981) suggests that the non-dominant hemisphere is a reserve of functions in case of regional failure and this functionality can be stimulated to delay the progression of degenerative disease. Furthermore, it is important to point out that when the overall

Table 7.2 Musical elements of assessment and examples of improvised playing

Musical elements of assessment	Examples of improvised playing
Testing of musical skills: rhythm, melody, harmony, dynamic, phrasing, articulation	Improvisations using rhythmic instruments (drum and cymbal) single or in combination
	Improvisations using melodic instruments
	Singing and playing folksongs with harmonic accompaniment
Cortical disorder testing: visio-spatial skills	Playing tuned percussion (metallophone, xylophone, chime bars) demanding precise movements
Cortical disorder testing: ability to perform complex motor tasks (including grip and right–left co-ordination)	Alternate playing of cymbal and drum using a beater in each hand
	Co-ordinated playing of cymbal and drum using a beater in each hand
	Co-ordinated playing of tuned percussion
Testing for progressive memory disintegration	The playing of short rhythmic and melodic phrases within the session, and in successive sessions
Motivation to sustain playing improvised music, to achieve musical goals and persevere in maintaining musical form	The playing of a rhythmic pattern deteriorates when unaccompanied by the therapist, as does the ability to complete a known melody, although tempo remains
'Intention' a feature of improvised musical playing	The patient exhibits the intention to play the piano from the onset of therapy and maintains this intent throughout the course of treatment
Concentration on the improvised playing and attention to the instruments	The patient loses concentration when playing, with qualitative loss in the musical playing and lack of precision in the beating of rhythmical instruments
Flexibility in musical (including instrumental) changes	Initially the musical playing is limited to a tempo of 120 beats per minute and a characteristic pattern, but this is responsive to change
Ability to play improvised music influenced by previous musical training	Although the patient has a musical background this is of help only when she perceives the musical playing; it is little influence in the improvised playing
Sensitive to small changes	Musical changes in tempo, dynamic, timbre and articulation which at first are missing are gradually developed
Ability to interpret musical context and relationship	The patient develops the ability to play in a musical dialogue with the therapist demanding both a refined musical perception and the ability of musical production

rhythmic pattern failed, the patient was able to maintain her beating in tempo. A similar situation applies in coma patients who cannot co-ordinate basic life pulses within a rhythmic context and thereby regain consciousness (Aldridge 1991b; Aldridge *et al.* 1990). We may need to address in future research the co-ordinating role of rhythm in human cognition and consciousness whether it be in persons who are losing cognitive abilities, or in persons who are attempting to gain cognitive abilities.

CHAPTER 8

Creative Music Therapy
A Last Resort?

Fraser Simpson

If I am no longer a woman, why do I still feel I'm one? If no longer worth holding, why do I crave it? If no longer sensual, why do I enjoy the soft texture of satin and silk against my skin? If no longer sensitive, why do moving song lyrics strike a responsive chord in me? My every molecule seems to scream out that I do, indeed, exist, and that existence must be valued by someone! Without someone to walk this labyrinth by my side, without the touch of a fellow-traveler who understands my need of self-worth, how can I endure the rest of this uncharted journey? (Diana Friel McGowin 1993, pp.123–124)

[Music] can lead or accompany the psyche through all conditions of inner experience, whether these be superficial and relatively common-place or profound and deeply personal. (Nordoff and Robbins 1971, p.15)

The wealth of literature that began to appear in the last decade of the twentieth century regarding the care and support of older people in our society has amounted to something of a revolution in the field of geron-tology. A new model of care has emerged that emphasizes the unique 'personhood' of all human beings (Goldsmith 1996; Kitwood 1997) based on the premise that despite the disintegrating effects of old age, and particu-larly of dementia, there remains always a sentient individual. This approach pays significantly greater attention to psychological and emotional needs than the medical establishment has traditionally offered in the past.

The onset of a dementing illness is often a double blow. In the first place, cognitive decline caused by progressive damage to the brain frequently creates the experience of ongoing trauma (Miesen and Jones 1997, p.152). The words that begin this chapter were written by somebody living in the early stages of dementia when articulate verbal expression was still possible, and constitute a moving personal testimony to the loneliness, desperation and terror that dementia often evokes. Yet cruelly, as the craving for comfort and support escalates, the possibility of addressing psychological and emotional needs by normal verbal means is systematically eroded, leaving the sufferer in a state of increasing isolation. As Miesen and Jones describe:

> A person with dementia gradually loses everything and slowly loses control of him or herself, becoming more and more what might be termed a 'displaced person'. The need to feel safe is activated, the need for proximity, the need to have and hold on to attachment figures. At the same time, the person experiences attachment figures as being less and less present. The diminishing capacity to keep new information in long-term store also causes the person with dementia slowly to lose awareness of the presence of, and emotional response from, attachment figures. Hence people with dementia can no longer find safety and well-being with friends, family or those around them. (Miesen and Jones 1997, p.149)

It is no wonder that an estimated one-third of people with dementia also show evidence of depression (Kitwood 1997, p.29). As the number of people in older age groups rises steadily, and with them the number of dementia sufferers, there is a pressing need for the development of non-verbal interventions which both counteract the isolation of a dementing illness and address emotional and psychological needs of the individual. This chapter aims to illustrate some of the principles of creative music therapy, with the belief that this particular form of music therapy offers significant and unique benefits in relation to these factors.

Creative music therapy

A pioneering way of using music clinically for therapeutic benefit was developed by Paul Nordoff and Clive Robbins in the 1950s and 1960s. Recognizing the universality of musical experience, they discovered that improvised music-making with children with developmental delay can be a powerful means of making contact, developing intercommunication skills, and facilitating both individual and social integration by combating isolation and emotional disturbance. They called this work *Creative Music Therapy* (Nordoff and Robbins 1977) to emphasize the central importance of active participation and spontaneity of the music improvised.

The principles of Nordoff and Robbins' approach, in which the development of a musical relationship between therapist and client through improvisation forms the vehicle of the therapy, has more recently been extended to work with adults in a variety of clinical areas including dementia care (Aldridge 1996; Ansdell 1995). While creative music therapy undoubtedly has much in common with other contemporary forms of music therapy, it does however contrast with approaches that use music to generate material for verbal elaboration, and those that consider improvised music to be unsuitable for people with dementia on the grounds that it may add to their confusion (Bright 1997, p.137). In the Nordoff–Robbins approach verbal dialogue is not generally considered to be central to the therapeutic process. Using improvisational structures the mutual participation of therapist and client creates a shared musical experience, even though no previous musical training or expertise is required of the client.

The case study that follows is the story of one man's journey in creative music therapy. The work took place in eight sessions over a period of three months and was recorded on audio and videotape to enable the music to be studied and analysed in detail.

Edward

At the age of 87, Edward entered a nursing home for people with advanced dementia. I began working with him there about a month after he arrived. Although every person has a unique story there are patterns which emerge, and some aspects of Edward's decline will undoubtedly be familiar to many people who have cared for a relative or friend through a dementing illness.

Edward had spent his working life as a skilled cabinet-maker. He was a placid man, and enjoyed good health right up until his late seventies when he began having heart problems. This led eventually to the insertion of a pacemaker, and it was when he was in his mid-eighties that the first signs of Alzheimer's disease began to appear. Initial confusion of faces and disorientation about the home progressed to more obvious loss of cognitive perception and speech; Edward began to spend all his time opening and closing doors, mumbling to himself and wandering at night.

For a while Edward's wife, to whom he had been married for sixty years, was able to continue caring for him at home but then Edward's personality seemed to change. He became aggressive and violent, sometimes ordering his wife around and even threatening to call the police. At the same time he clung to her and became extremely anxious when left on his own. The time came, inevitably, when Edward's wife, who herself was becoming frail, could no longer cope. Following a lengthy assessment procedure it was decided that Edward's needs would best be met by placing him in a residential home where his wife would be able to visit him regularly. To reduce his agitation Edward was prescribed a tranquillizer; he became withdrawn, spending increasing amounts of time in a state of apathy and passivity, usually not getting out of bed before 11.00 a.m. and then sitting inactively for the rest of the day. When I met him, Edward seemed thoroughly depressed, disempowered by his loss of independence. His speech was reduced to short mumbled phrases that were often hard to understand, and similarly it was difficult for him to make sense of other people's words. Furthermore walking was also a great difficulty, aggravated by his loss of motivation.

Phase One – meeting Edward in music – sessions 1–3

I went to see Edward in the sitting room to invite him for his first session. As was to be the case on most subsequent occasions, he was initially reluctant to move, being comfortably settled in an arm-chair, and without the use of normal language I could not explain in a way that made any sense to him where I wanted us to go. Eventually with grumbling effort he rose to his feet. 'Where are we going?' he mumbled in bewilderment as we walked slowly down the corridor. 'What's it all for?'

As we reached the music therapy room Edward paused and looked around at the array of instruments laid out: a drum and cymbal, metallophone, various small percussion instruments and a piano in the corner. 'I don't play any of these'. He sounded utterly dejected, and the words expressed his attitude of defeat to the trial his life had become. Helping him to a chair, I put the drum in front of him and demonstrated with a few beats how to play it. 'Would you like to try this, Edward?' 'Me? No... I can't... my brain's too short'. Although his words were confused, they conveyed with singular clarity his present state of mind and experience of dementia.

I began to improvise at the piano quietly, trying a few different musical styles. Edward looked interested but did not make any sound. Out of the corner of my eye I noticed his foot tapping in time with the music; clearly he was engaged at some level. I decided to play an old music-hall tune to see whether Edward would show any recognition, and chose 'Daisy Bell', a well-known popular song from the era of Edward's youth. Immediately Edward sprang into life. 'No, no, not too loud!…that's it, smoothly…it's not slowly enough…that's it!' As I adapted my playing in accordance with Edward's instructions his hands began to move expressively in the air, giving further indication of how he wanted the music played. 'Smoothly…that's better'. Then, as we reached the end of a phrase he tried to demonstrate with his voice how the last interval should sound. I repeated it back to him and he sang it once again. Effortlessly Edward had been drawn into active music-making.

After this I began to move out from the song: it had served its purpose and now I wanted to explore Edward's own musical creativity. He was still making animated hand movements, and as I continued to play they became more decisive. He seemed to be conducting me, totally absorbed in the music as if he were actually playing the piano himself. A few minutes earlier I had placed a tambourine on his lap, and he gradually now began to tap it very quietly, perfectly in time with the music. Holding the instrument in one hand, his playing became a little louder as his confidence grew. He started to use his fingers separately, again creating the feeling in me that he was experiencing the piano music I played as coming from his own hands. And in a sense this was precisely what was happening since I was attempting to create music – it was a delicate, nimble waltz – that harmonized with the quality of his tapping.

But Edward eventually seemed to tire, and I was perhaps a little too enthusiastic in my attempts to keep him playing. 'No,' he said, 'you're miles in front of me'. I tried slowing the pace of the music but Edward clearly wanted me to stop. 'No…it's impossible for me to get up…I'm coming down'. I brought the music to a close and helped Edward to his feet. 'It's been good to spend this time with you, Edward'. 'Yes,' he replied slowly, 'I was going to say the same'. Despite the way the improvisation had ended he clearly took away a positive experience of the session. I was struck by the contrast between Edward's initial mood and the music that had emerged, giving him a very different experience to his familiar state of apathy.

As I greeted Edward for the second time a week later he gave no indication of recognition. This was to happen every week throughout the duration of our work and was of interest since it became gradually apparent over the weeks that at a musical level some memory of the sessions was being retained. Yet he did not seem to remember my appearance. On this occasion Edward was rather sleepy. It was mid-morning and he had not been up for long. It was some weeks before I realized that mornings were not his best time, and took to making sure that his sessions were scheduled for the afternoon. This time I went straight in with a song. It was another well-known one, 'A Nightingale Sang in Berkeley Square', which had a dreamy quality that seemed to resonate with Edward's disposition that day. Edward began to hum along, tunefully but in a rather half-hearted way. Before we reached the end, his eyes had closed and he was dozing peacefully. Gently nudging him awake, I played 'The White Cliffs of Dover', which Edward recognized as well. However, the same thing happened again. Yet, even as Edward drifted into slumber, he continued to murmur the tones of the song as I played. It was as though the music was being experienced at a subconscious level, accompanying and permeating his whole being.

The following week, in session 3, we moved into a new level of experience altogether. Edward came into the room wide awake, and did not want to sit in the usual chair beside the piano, despite my prompting. Instead, as I sat at the piano, he stood behind me with an arm on the back of the chair. For over half an hour we played and sang through a selection of old songs, including the ones that had been introduced in the previous two sessions. Edward sang in a different way today, with purpose and definition, absorbed by his engagement in the music we were making together. His singing was all wordless vocalization; it seemed almost as if the music liberated him from the struggle with words, and in fact Edward continued to sing in this way throughout our subsequent sessions.[1] Now he sang with great feeling, and was clearly investing emotional energy in the music, as the tears welling up in his eyes signified. We were like performers on a stage, and there was a sense of deep connection between us.[2] It certainly was incredible that somebody so unsteady on his legs could remain standing for such a long time without tiring. In this way the music enabled Edward to move beyond the confines of his day-to-day existence.

Reflections on Phase One

In these opening sessions Edward's innate musicality allowed a true 'meeting' to take place within the musical context. There is a peculiarly intimate quality in music that can enable two people to *mean the same thing in the same moment* in a way that is impossible with words, and which can transcend the limitations of a disability or illness.

We had relied quite heavily on pre-composed music. Clive Robbins (Aigen 1996, p.20) has described with a lovely metaphor how a song can act like a boat, enabling people to literally 'step into it and sail into music'. While the Nordoff–Robbins approach is rooted in improvised music as a basis for interaction and exploration it also recognizes and makes use of the power of song to elicit musical engagement. However, what I now wanted was to work to make his musical presence more actively creative, so that rather than my merely accompanying or playing 'for' him, he would be able to participate at an interactive level. Such work requires fine tuning of the music therapist's clinical judgement: in that first session as Edward faltered towards the end I realized that there can be a thin line between 'enabling' and 'disabling' a person in music therapy.[3] Too little, and the client has no starting-point to grasp hold of; too much, and the client is easily overpowered. In this case Edward's experience of his dementia must have come flooding back as the music threatened to overwhelm him. I would need to take great care to listen and respond to what Edward was telling me through his music.

The loss of ability to make choices is one of the pernicious consequences of dementia, and quality care focuses on enabling sufferers to retain as much control over their lives as possible. Edward's reluctance to make the journey down to the music therapy room evoked conflicting feelings in me even though I believed that he was not specifically rejecting music therapy. As I urged him to join me I was torn between his preference to remain where he was comfortable and my awareness that music therapy had something of value to offer him.

Phase Two – a deepening relationship – sessions 4–6

In his life outside music therapy, Edward's level of functioning was deteriorating quite rapidly. Even since our first session I had noticed that his speech had become less coherent, and the perceptions of the nursing team at the home supported this observation. As is so often the case in the presence of a dementing illness, it was difficult to know whether this degeneration was a direct result of neurological impairment, or whether depression might also be a contributing factor. In view of the rapidity of his decline since coming to the nursing home, the latter seemed likely. In music therapy, however, I was seeing a different side to Edward, and it was in session 4 that he began really to improvise for the first time.

Once again, Edward moved from the sitting room to the music therapy room with reluctance, grumbling unintelligibly to himself as he shuffled falteringly down the corridor. We opened with a couple of familiar songs, in which he joined me rather half-heartedly, approximating the tune under his breath. However, as he sang Edward began to take notice of the drum that was standing beside him, perhaps attracted by its shiny metal rim, and started to fiddle with it. It was the first time that he had shown interest in an instrument since his first session, and I judged that this might be a good time to encourage him to play again. Placing the drum in front of Edward, I produced a stick and hit the drum three times to demonstrate how to play. Immediately, to my surprise, he answered vocally, repeating the three sounds in the key of the music I had just been playing: 'da da da' (Figure 8.1, bar 1). I repeated the sequence on the drum, but Edward was quiet again, so I tried to put the drum-stick into his hand. 'Take the stick, Edward'. Then again in response to this he repeated the three notes (Figure 8.1, bar 3). This time I played the sequence on the piano, matching his pitch. He continued to respond vocally, rather than taking the stick, and we moved into an interactive dialogue with Edward adapting both pitch and rhythmic patterns in accordance with what I played (Figure 8.1, bars 4–9).

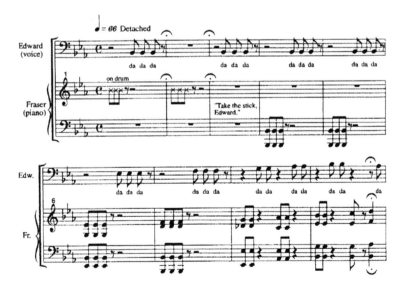

Figure 8.1

As we continued, Edward became more playful, responding to the musical idiom that was emerging and using it creatively. As always, he sang without words. The music in Figure 8.2 occurred about two minutes after the music in Figure 8.1, and is an example of how the improvisational context enabled us to engage mutually through our music-making. The use of inevitable harmonic sequences facilitated his participation, although I did not impose them as a premeditated intervention; rather we found them together.

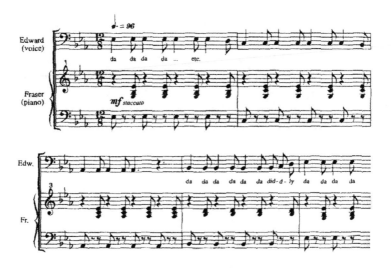

Figure 8.2

Edward was still holding the stick I had placed in his hand, and he began to tap it lightly but crisply on the side of the piano beside which he was sitting. Rhythmically he was not too precise at first, but he obviously liked the sensation, and I tried to base what I was playing on the sounds he made. He clearly registered the connection, as Figure 8.3 illustrates: I began to leave 'obvious' pauses in the music, and Edward responded by filling those pauses, and so a musical rapport was established. The effect of this was that Edward's playing became more intentional and stable, although he continued to have difficulty playing in a precise tempo.

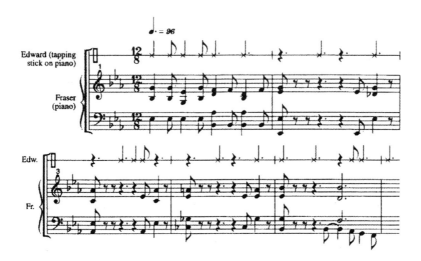

Figure 8.3

When he had been tapping the piano for a couple of minutes I motioned towards the drum with my hand and Edward took the cue, beginning now to play it in a similar kind of way. His beating was quiet and uncertain as he adjusted to the new experience, yet he was listening intently with full concentration on the musical interaction. As I made tempo changes, speeding up or slowing down, Edward followed me with considerable accuracy. With an irrepressible sense of purpose he was totally engrossed in the experience we were sharing. I noticed with interest that a growing contrast seemed to be developing between Edward's lack of external awareness and his increasing musical engagement: he gave almost no eye contact and seemed hardly aware of me as a person in the room, yet as a musical presence he could relate to me directly and intimately.

In the next two sessions Edward appeared musically to be more distant again. Perhaps it was the time of day, but his involvement was less intense. Verbally he had no intelligible language at all, although he mumbled to himself: the rapidity of his decline was obvious and striking. Yet in session 5 he also seemed to consolidate his achievements of the previous session, leaving me with the feeling that he must be retaining some memory of the sessions even if he never seemed to recognize me. Initially Edward had difficulty connecting the drum-stick to the drum, not really managing to produce a coherent beat, and appeared to lose interest as a result. I offered him a maraca as a different way of making a sound; he accepted this and immediately began to tap the drum with it. Playing the piano I adopted his tempo and followed his lead, slowing and speeding up with him. Edward's playing was almost inaudible and I had to work hard to scale my music down to match the quality of his.

Edward maintained this for nearly ten minutes, even though he seemed terribly tired that day. As he settled into the music he became gradually louder, able to imitate simple rhythmic patterns, although anything sudden or unexpected seemed to confuse him and lead him to trail off. He seemed to need me to function more in an accompanying role, rather than to present anything too challenging. In a similar way to the first session Edward appeared to experience my piano-playing as emanating directly from himself: for example, when I improvised melodic figures as in Figure 8.4 in time to Edward's beat, he spontaneously began to move his hand from side to side on the drum to fit the music, as though he himself were playing the melody. Unlike session 1, however, he had now become far more actively involved in the actual act of musical creation.

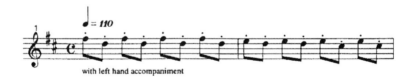

Figure 8.4

The following week in session 6, Edward seemed even more fragile. As with our second meeting a few weeks earlier, it was a morning session and he drifted in and out of sleep as I played the piano. I offered some familiar tunes again, with which Edward periodically hummed along quietly, but he did not look at the instruments. There was no intention in his music or his being; at the time I felt he was slipping away.

Reflections on Phase Two

As Edward joined me in musical dialogue something of significance was at work. Although he had become severely impaired in his ability to interact spontaneously with others, he had not lost the will to do so, and the simplest of musical devices was offering him the possibility to remake this connection with the outside world. It is in this realm that the value of creative music therapy becomes apparent. Music is improvised not *for* but *with* the client, who participates in the creation of something which is at once both communicative and expressive. As the darkening isolation of dementia descends this can provide individuals with confirmation that they are, indeed, alive, and that relatedness with other people is still possible.

The length of time that Edward was able to remain absorbed in the musical experience was also significant. I marvelled at the capacity of music to act as such a powerful motivator, enabling him to concentrate on the activity for probably far longer than he would now be able to sustain in other situations. Music manifests in time, and it seems that for people like Edward, for whom dementia disturbs the natural sense of time-flow and event-sequences, music can provide an experience of continuity and orientation. Ansdell (1995) has described how

> the order of music can recall a sense of order when the self is threatened by the chaos of the external world or from the disordering effects of illness or handicap...music can provide a more solid world than does everyday reality. (Ansdell 1995, p.134)

The power of music in this way evokes a kind of 'recall' into centredness and integration.

Phase Three – new departures – sessions 7–8

When I saw Edward a week later for his seventh session, I sensed a renewed purpose in his music-making. Looking physically more frail and walking with greater difficulty, his engagement in music seemed almost to defy his decline. Edward took the drum-stick between his thumb and forefinger and began to play the drum with control and ease, as well as with greater clarity and purpose than previously. Figure 8.5 comes from about eleven minutes into the session and illustrates how he responded to phrase-lengths and simple structural devices to enjoy a communicative musical dialogue, rather like the one in session 4 (Figure 8.3), except that he was now playing more confidently and coherently.

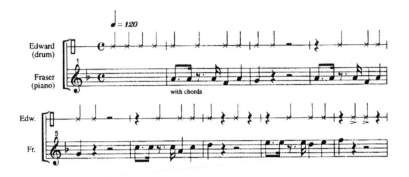

Figure 8.5

Later in the session Edward put down the stick and we moved into song. There was a quality in his voice that I had not heard before – an expressive flexibility and commitment to the musical 'performance' that we were rendering together. I selected a traditional song with a rather slow and sober nature, 'The Old Folks at Home', that he clearly knew well, and which called out from him the expression of something quite deep. Edward discovered a remarkable new versatility in his range of pitch; singing at times in 'falsetto' voice he soared up an octave over my piano accompaniment. Between verses or recapitulations of the melody I improvised short phrases with my voice that he answered, also in improvisation, resulting in an intimate vocal dialogue that we had not found together before.

The song reached a natural end and Edward took up the drum-stick again. This time he held the stick in the middle, over the drum so that both ends of the stick were able to touch the metal rim on opposite sides of the drum. This produced a clicking sound, and with a skilful wrist action Edward created a lively 'tap-dancing' effect, as indicated in Figure 8.6. Again he was responsive to the music that I invented to accompany him, he listened intently and deftly altered his rhythm appropriately.

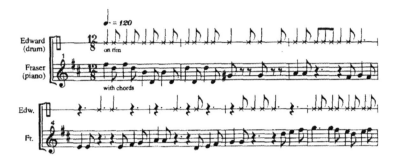

Figure 8.6

When I went to see Edward in the sitting room for his eighth session I found him repeating a single phrase to himself. It was the first time for a few weeks that I had heard him say anything I could comprehend. He was saying quite simply, 'I can't do anything...I can't do anything'. After much encouragement he eventually summoned the strength and motivation to make the walk down to the music therapy room.

Today I began to play the song 'Blue Moon'. Edward immediately began to sing with me and, like the previous session, he expressed complete commitment to the music we were making, both in the tone quality of his singing and the creativity with which he participated. Again between repetitions of the tune I offered short improvised phrases which he answered with ease and natural musicality. Figure 8.7, in which a brief portion of this interaction is transcribed, begins with Edward's singing of the well-known tune, which I supported with a light chordal accompaniment (not shown). As he reached the end of the verse (bar 8) I entered with a short improvised phrase, thus initiating an interactive dialogue. Edward's voice moved up into the 'falsetto' register as he responded to me with unconstrained and charming engagement. There was complete mutuality in this music, and it felt almost as though his cares were literally dropping away from him as he sang.

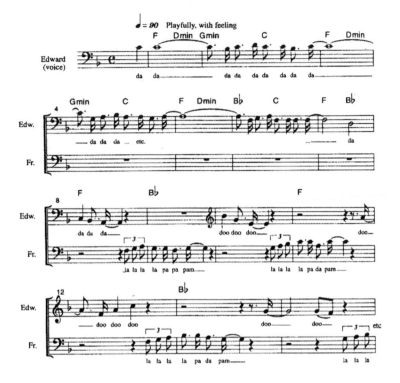

Figure 8.7

We sustained this kind of intense interaction for a period of over five minutes, moving periodically away from and back to the tune of 'Blue Moon'. At times Edward's delight in his vocal dexterity led to the spontaneous evolution of extended phrases such as the one in Figure 8.8.

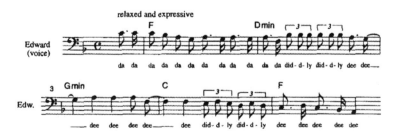

Figure 8.8

Towards the end Edward suddenly stopped singing quite abruptly, and rising from his chair he moved unsteadily across the room. I continued to play, wondering what was happening: had he had enough and was wishing to leave? Then my fears were quelled as Edward, standing at first quite still, began to swing his arms at his side with the music, and then he was singing again, immersed in the musical experience. In fact Edward was dancing; it was an electrifying and unforgettable moment. Here was a man who appeared to be defying the illness that threatened his very existence, a man who in one sense was utterly alive and well.

Reflections on Phase Three

That we talk about playing music is of course no accident, for music in its essence is indeed a kind of play, albeit at times of a sophisticated nature. Thus among the benefits that creative music therapy offers is the opportunity to encounter oneself anew as spontaneous, creative and joyful – aspects of human experience which it would be difficult to see somebody in Edward's state of health encountering in any other way. In these two final sessions Edward's capacity for play acquired a new clarity in our improvised music-making.

Yet there is also something about the nature of music that expresses the ambivalence of human feeling, so that both joy and sadness can coexist in the same musical phrase, as in life. It felt as though Edward and I had explored a whole range of emotions together in this third phase of the therapy. This is not the place to discuss the meaning of emotion in music, an inexhaustible subject for debate, except to say that music is clearly far more than the expression of specific transitory mood-states that may affect us at one time or another. As philosopher Susanne Langer said, music is 'Not the symptomatic expression of feelings that beset the composer but a symbolic expression of the forms of sentience as he understands them' (Langer 1953, p.28). Thus creative music therapy, being based on the use of improvised music, primarily offers a space not for cathartic release of habitually experienced feelings and emotions, but for exploration of unpredictable and different ones; it is a space where people 'stuck' in a pathological state such as depression may have a new experience of themselves and therefore a new experience of life itself.

As Edward sang and danced, it seemed to me in that moment that however devastating and depersonalizing the effects of a dementing illness, however convincingly a person seems to drift away into the realms of 'unbeing', there is yet something inside that remains intact, a spirit that constitutes the vital essence of personhood. Music, the 'Quickening Art', as Kant described it (Ansdell 1995, p.81), stands perhaps unique in its capacity to make contact with, and give life to, this spirit.

Afterthoughts

Kitwood (1997, pp.81–84) proposes a five-fold model of care that he believes encompasses the main psychological needs of people with dementia. The five areas he identifies are: comfort, attachment, inclusion, occupation and identity. These areas overlap and come together, he suggests, to form one all-encompassing need – LOVE. The example of Edward described in this chapter has shown, I hope, how well creative music therapy resonates with this model, offering:

- comfort, because music's consoling power can reach depths of the psyche that far surpass the level that can be reached by words;

- attachment, because the communicative potential of improvised music means that relationship may continue unimpeded by verbal losses;

- inclusion, because the music is created spontaneously and is incomplete without the individual's personal contribution;

- occupation, because participative music-making concentrates the mind, encouraging the development of skill and imagination;

- identity, because to experience oneself in dynamic relationship with another reinforces a sense of self that transcends the debilitation of a mind-dissolving disease.

Creative music therapy in fact brings a whole new meaning to one of Shakespeare's most famous lines: in a very real sense music is indeed the food of love.

A further understanding of creative music therapy in the context of dementia care may be drawn from an extract of John Daniel's (1996) autobiographical account of his mother's slow decline and eventual death from Alzheimer's disease. He writes:

I wish I could have provided her with a ritual, a ceremony, some form or path for approaching death by which the troubles and longings of her spirit could have expressed themselves...I wish she could have cried and

laughed and worked it all through and come to something, to a final *Yes,
this is what my life has been, and it's all right*. (Daniel 1996, p.93)

Ritual may seem to have become an anachronism in contemporary western
society, although even our recent ancestors lived lives richly imbued with rit-
ualistic practices both sacred and secular. The great spiritual traditions from
all parts of the world evolved elaborate rites of passage, and point to a
profound need in the human psyche for ritual as a means of finding meaning
and healing. Writers such as James Roose-Evans (1994) testify to the steady
resurgence of interest today in creating rituals to mark life's significant
events, including preparation for death. But how can people who are robbed
of their cognitive faculties create and participate in meaningful ritual?

As a space where, unencumbered by words, emotions may well up and
find expression, meaning may be shared, and life may be truly *lived*, creative
music therapy can, I believe, facilitate such evolution of personal and spontaneous ritual. For Edward, I cannot say for certain what his experience may
have been in our work together, but I can say that it was a privilege for me to
participate, if only briefly, in his journey; and as we shared those moments it
seemed to me that somewhere, at some deep level, in that final session he was
able to say: *'Yes, this is what my life has been, and it's all right'*.

Notes

1   Interestingly, for other patients with whom I have worked the reverse of this has often
    been the case. People who have seemingly lost all verbal capacity as their dementia
    progresses have instantly remembered and reproduced the words of songs upon
    hearing the familiar tune associated with those words.

2   The concept of music therapy as performance is explored by Aldridge (1996,
    pp.20–30) and Ansdell (1995, pp.217–219). They appeal not to a conventional idea
    of performance where an audience is present, but to the idea of dynamic participation
    in a musical act as opposed to passive receipt of a musical experience.

3   This distinction between 'enabling' and 'disabling' interventions in music therapy is
    explored in detail by Richard Thompson (1997).

CHAPTER 9

Remembering and Forgiving

Susan Weber

An older generation of Germans is dying out. There is ample research and documentation on Holocaust survivors and their children (Bar-On 1989; Holliday 1995). There are even groups working together in Germany bringing members of the next generation of Jews and Germans together (Merritt 1998). However, research is just beginning to emerge on what happened on a personal level in Germany during and after the war (Goldhagen 1996; Owings 1995). It is interesting that the origins of so much music therapy came out of the aftermath of the Second World War (Mandel 1991), but only a small part of the needy were offered help. The rest were overlooked and/or forgotten.

This generation experienced war. They were perpetrators, victims or heroes. They went through prison camps. Those at home, after being bombed into oblivion, had to immediately start rebuilding a mostly destroyed country. Soon after, a part of the population had to deal with living under communism. Although to the outer world they resumed a normal life, the inner reality was often quite different. They often led a life of 'chronic sorrow' (Martinson 1992) built on guilt, shame, remorse, isolation and depression. The guilt may be related to concrete situations. Situations that were beyond control. Some issues have been left unfinished or unresolved. Guilt is an element of depression. Depression may also involve feelings of remorse, isolation, self-loathing and the eventual confrontation of one's own mortality (Ortiz 1997). These are not 'diseases' for medical intervention. Few even thought about therapy in the post-war period. None was offered. The population was forced to rely on themselves. Silence and repression from all sides became an effective means of survival. There was no concept of post-trauma stress in this post-Second World War period, and even less so for a population seen as collaborators and often as perpetrators.

Psychological profile

The following is mostly based on my personal contact and observations with older Germans who have been my patients, with German contemporaries and conversations with clinic and hospice staff. These sources report that most of their parents and friends never said anything about these experiences until around the age of 75 years, then some of them began to talk. Sometimes grandparents talked about their war experiences, more readily talking to their grandchildren than to their own children (Roberts 1994). However, they normally related their experiences without any emotional content – like a depersonalized adventure story. Their children and grandchildren were shocked as they had no idea of what exactly their parents or grandparents did or went through, good or bad. It became a subtle, unspoken inheritance.

As most soldiers, the Germans felt like broken men after the war. However, many of these men believed they were fighting for something noble or felt they had no choice (Merritt 1998). The very young ones drafted towards the end of the war experienced an additional terror as there were often other German soldiers behind them with pointed rifles, making sure they fought. Rather than allow themselves to feel their own pain of disillusionment, they 'turned to stone' and became tough (Merritt 1998). Many of them survived the additional shame of years of imprisonment and the atrocities in the Russian prisoner of war camps. To cope they became even more emotionally repressed and even more wooden. Although this may have been life saving, it also takes a great deal of energy to suppress initially, until this suppression becomes habitual. Habits, however, are hard to break and they affect other parts of our expressive life. Thus we have a generation of men unable to express the unspoken, which later had a significant effect upon their family lives.

Victims and members of the resistance also remained silent. I can only imagine the feelings towards those men and women 'of conscience' from those with such terrible guilt. Also the German resistance and the very active Jewish one (Suhi 1975) were kept hushed up. These people often have a very heroic attitude about their illness and impending death, such as 'This isn't so bad' or 'I can handle it', or on the other hand, 'No desire, nor energy, left to fight again'.

The nursing staff in the hospice have noticed that former perpetrators of atrocities do not like to be touched and really shy away from physical contact. The necessary nursing, and especially being bathed, can be excruciating for them. It is not uncommon for their bodies to become almost rigid. Several nurses have asked me for tapes to play during their baths, solely for muscle relaxation. Also, if the men are actively talking about their part in atrocities, and this does happen, I notice that the nurses start having as little to do with them as possible – just the basic necessities in contrast to the amount of time they normally spend with patients. Interestingly, these patients usually do not want my services as compared to the heroes and victims. I assume they do not want any emotional stimulation or to have to deal with the feelings that might come up.

I have never spoken with a female perpetrator or at least no one has ever admitted it to me. The women I have cared for usually grew up in an innocent world which turned into hell. They were young women, many newly married, often pregnant. Suddenly, their husbands were gone, and they were trying to stay alive, find food and fuel, in and out of bomb shelters, losing everything, running from soldiers to avoid rape (many were raped and not just once) and murder, and trying somehow to keep going. They did not know if they would ever see their husbands again, and were often resettled far from home without any extended family. Many of them had no idea of what had actually been going on in Germany and when they found out, their horror and shame was overwhelming. One told me, 'When I saw what had happened I thought that I would have to kill myself in order to offer some atonement. I was so ashamed to be a German'. At the same time she was pregnant, had one small son and no idea where her husband was. He appeared shortly after the war but looking like a living skeleton rather than a fully grown man. So she nursed him back to health, delivered her baby and then got on with the business of literally building a place to live. Nobody had any time to mourn and when there finally was some time, nobody dared bring it up openly. This somewhat supports the old Teutonic tradition: 'You must be strong and not show your feelings. This kind of strength is something to be proud of'.

The female victims, especially those who were raped, and many were by whomever happened to be passing through, initially tell me that I should not play and waste all my time just for them. They have lived with great shame and do not feel worthy of special care and have usually been great caregivers themselves. Their body language is rather reserved, pulled back. They have been stuck in denial, guilt and shame and have often suffered a deep inner loneliness and, oddly enough, the feelings that they may have been the only one who went through such things. Many have held themselves distant from their families and perhaps never experienced real intimacy. This may also

have led them to become very self-reliant. A great part of this defence is now
stripped away because of their dependency on others for physical needs
(Gilbert 1977).

I often wonder if the rebuilding of Germany was subconsciously a
healing ritual, letting out some of that pent-up energy and that is why it progressed so quickly. You can fall asleep after that kind of extreme manual
labour. Being the aggressors also led to the loss of a positive personal and
national identity. It became very uncomfortable on the world stage to be
identified as a German, and they became too ashamed, or guilty, to be their
real selves. Some are still confused about the difference between nationalism
and patriotism. Even the younger generation can barely sing the German
national anthem and often do not know the text. So here is an entire population who undoubtedly went through post-traumatic stress – with all that
involves, freezing emotionally, nightmares, misdirected anger and often
undisclosed self-loathing.

Healing inner wounds

Most cancer patients experience a strong sense of loss of control. For these
older Germans, the disease, the treatment and everything associated have just
been another repetition of the past, so to speak. In addition, this group has
felt out of control most of their lives and they are now faced with the final
lack of control – death. Certainly in order to heal any of this inner turmoil,
they have to be able to start to feel again.

As in any hospice, we are no longer dealing in healing physical ailments;
rather, much of my healing work deals with these inner wounds of hate, guilt,
shame and resentment. For some patients, their impending death is actually a
comfort because all of this will finally be over. For others, it is terrifying
because they fear that which may come. As with other dying patients, they
share the common need to review either the totality or a portion of their past
lives.

These Germans grew up amidst a very rich musical life at home. Many
played instruments and sang together. It was something that was beautiful,
fun and certainly a positive representation of their culture. Some of my older
German friends have told me how they sang themselves sane in prison camps.
They are usually the ones who were aged between 16 and 20. An enormous
number of them went back to playing their instruments or singing in

choruses. Perhaps this was another survival mechanism and offered some emotional release and the feeling of belonging to a group.

As a musician and psychologist I see music being a decisive factor, having a stronger healing effect than just talking alone. I have no idea where the role of psychologist or music therapist begins or ends (Aldridge 1993c). The artist in me is concerned with offering these patients a beautiful experience and the psychologist in offering some help in finding some relief and the gentle companionship that results from the music alone or the talking.

Music is a familiar medium and can be a springboard towards discussing this inner pain (Sears 1966) that many of them have never expressed, although they are often desperate to find some relief from the real, or imagined, guilt. The terrible personal suffering is very real. These are some of my most important moments as a music therapist – helping people express this sadness or shame, start the process of forgiving, ask for forgiveness and reconnect to their own gentle feelings. I sense this as beginning the inner process of healing old wounds, finding personal and spiritual resources, some of which they may never have been aware of, and easing the process of dying. I have learned that even though the thought goes through my mind – this person is going to be here for only a little while – there is no rule that you cannot make friends when a person is dying, helping them feel included (Lochner and Stevenson 1988). Perpetrators and victims often had no real intimacy, physical or emotional, and they are afraid of it. The non-verbal aspect of music is so well suited for these people. Making ourselves under-stood to one another can be a very complex issue (Mohacsy 1995) and music can simplify it.

Creativity is considered to be an integral part of music-making and the question can arise: 'Is creativity possible with the dying?' *Webster's New Ency-clopedic Dictionary* (1993) defines creating as 'bringing something about'. So what is it that I want to bring about? I would say that creativity in my work is following my intuition and seeking the music that can bring about a safe environment where the patient can just be. Where we can be together. In this little time left of life, perhaps we can re-establish some other appropriate coping mechanisms. The patient can share with me whatever they wish to share, and perhaps resolve some of it, find peace with their loved ones and prepare to leave with greater ease.

Except those staying for pain management and then returning home, the patients usually spend the last two weeks of their lives in the hospice and are extremely weak. Receptive music is in the foreground. They simply do not have the strength or desire to be actively involved. I begin by offering them a compact disc player and the music they would like to hear. I also ask them if they would like me to play for them, stressing that I will play only the music they want to hear. The hospice has a piano on wheels which I can push into their rooms, or I use a small 'Veeh Harp'. The majority request the piano. In this weaker state, they do not care so much for improvisation but tend to prefer well-known music or pieces with a marked structure.

When I begin to work with patients, they are initially looking for a certain distracting element and always relaxation. A lot of classical music is requested at the beginning, especially Mozart. I expect that this high selection of classical music is also cultural. There is also not quite the same category of religious music in Germany as in the United States or Britain and this classical music may be a substitute.

I have found that when a patient has no specific musical request, and many do not, at least in the beginning, it is more beneficial to start with music that they do not necessarily have any memories or emotional ties with. Music that has a lilting melody and gentle rhythm. In Germany I am free to use the lovely folksongs from England, Wales, Scotland and Ireland. Most of the patients say that they sound vaguely familiar but they seldom bring up any concrete memories. They enjoy them, learn to fall back on the music and relax. I find them excellent for calming heart and breathing rates, and they are also very popular with family members. This music allows me an initial contact that is non-threatening, especially with these people who have been extremely threatened. They often seem able to stay in the present and enjoy the actual moment – the 'hear and now' (Ortiz 1997, p.243). We both breathe more easily and relax; I sense the patient's trust.

I strongly feel that it is important to reintroduce aesthetic experiences and genuine beauty to people, especially those who because of their disease and past experiences may have been without such experiences. A retreat from such experiences may have served to anaesthetize them from so much abuse (Knill 1995). It is my responsibility to create the presence of beauty and love, possibly turning the aesthetic experience into a therapeutic one, if the patient is willing. At the same time, the music offers me a psychological buffer as this whole issue is not particularly palatable, nor easy, for me to deal with. This beauty and love certainly makes it easier for me to cope with what I am often confronted with. I can protect myself behind it or the aesthetic aspect mellows it out, offering me emotional release. I am not looking for sensational histories and when they are told a part of me wants to scream, 'I really do not want to hear this'. Again the music can dissolve some of that horror or disgust or the thought, 'Can we human beings really sink that low?' It also allows me and my patients the possibility to respond with a 'Yes', but we can also soar as high as the beauty in the music. Music is an aesthetic tradition, especially in Germany, and will evoke an aesthetic response. This aesthetic musical history is something positive, to be proud of, and can be another aspect of the healing component. In this way the music also keeps me from distancing myself too far. I cannot be superficial and open my heart, keep cool and still play beautifully.

I notice that it often seems more natural starting up a conversation after I have first played for a patient. I usually ask them to tell me about themselves. The conversation can go in any direction from talking about the pictures of their grandchildren, favourite pastimes, their own musical experiences, what gave their life meaning and whatever else they may want to discuss. The music is very varied and often their requests change with their moods. At this point, almost no one asks to hear German folk music. That happens later.

The ritual

Sometimes patients are able to recognize that old thought and feeling habits are no longer necessary and understand that they can be replaced with new possibilities. This may be made easier by creating a ritual (Achterberg, Dossey and Kolkmeier 1994). Rituals can be empowering (Dossey 1993) connecting us back to our inner resources. There are few rituals that do not include music.

Breathing more easily, deep relaxation and visualization can set the healing in motion. Music supports all of these processes. It can bring up memories and long-buried emotions and yet offer a continuing comfort at the same time. This can be the beginning of a ritual that goes through the telling of the event, remembering the pain, and possibly crying it out. The patient can then start to forgive and let go of the hate, shame or resentment and possibly begin to approach the idea of reconciliation (Augsburger 1996). A ritual cannot eradicate what happened but together with the music it can offer a container, allowing the repressed pain to take a form which can be released and resolved.

Forgiveness

Healing these inner wounds is going to include a lot of forgiveness. Asking forgiveness of those we hurt, forgiving those who hurt us and finally forgiving ourselves. Forgiveness is a matter of the heart and along with music, I use the following type of visualization. It has proven to be a good starting place.

After starting with general relaxing music or a relaxing text, I begin the following:

> Allow yourself to see an image emerge of a person, dead or alive, who brings up negative feelings. And, as that image is forming, notice your heart and the area around your heart opening. Allow the image of the person who brings up these unhappy feelings to enter your heart centre. From the spaciousness of your heart centre hold the picture of this person as you repeat, 'For anything that may have happened between us in the past, remembered or not, in thoughts, words, or actions which caused one of us pain – I forgive you'.
>
> And as you do this, notice any change in any of your negative feelings – the hardness becoming softer, resentment turning to understanding, and a gradual acceptance of this change. If any thoughts intrude, return to the image of the person and your new feelings. If unpleasant body sensations arise, let them be and continue concentrating on the changes watching – noticing – feeling – all changes – opening your heart, for this moment. Just continue to focus on the image of the person – speaking from your heart – releasing your negative feelings – pain – forgiving yourself – forgiving others [Achterberg *et al.* 1994, p.276]. You may want to ask forgiveness of your family members and close friends, perhaps for acting reserved or holding back your positive feelings because you, yourself, were too afraid to feel. You may do this now. The person does not have to be here with you.
>
> When you feel you have forgiven and let go of the resentment, say, 'And now I forget it. It is over. I do not have to carry this with me anymore. I am free to go forward. I am free to leave'.

A total release may not be immediate and the process may be repeated. The result is sometimes, if possible, that the patient will talk to the other person who has been hurt or has caused injury. In other words, healing can begin to take place in a relationship too as well as for the patient. The short amount of time before dying and an intense desire for relief often quickens the process.

Music, along with this type of visualization emphasizing forgiveness and inner peace, may also restore hope and allow patients to rebuild an inner, more spiritual reality and also rediscover the many things, large and small, they have to be grateful for (Linn 1977).

Many of these people become very focused on a material world, blocking out the emotional and spiritual one. They felt spiritually abandoned asking: 'What kind of God could let such things happen?' They are about to leave a material world and body and enter a different level of existence. Rediscovering and reconnecting to an inner reality is significant for the process of dying. If palliative care is concerned with relieving suffering, it is this existential suffering, as well as pain, that needs to be addressed.

As Larry Dossey says in conversation with Norman Goldberg:

> Music helps people to identify and find meaning in their lives by becoming more sensitive to something more powerful and majestic than themselves – whether called 'the spiritual', God, Goddess, the Absolute or something else. Music and the arts help us fine tune our lives. (Goldberg 1998, pp.41–42)

After the visualization I play again and use the music to further the sense of release and often produce deep sleep. This whole process may also help patients attend to that which they will leave behind, establish a right relationship with what they do between now and the final hour, no matter what the past was, or create a ceremony for the final hour and beyond.

Family

When a person is dying the family find themselves in a crisis situation where the joys and regrets of the past, the demands of the present and the fears of the future are all brought into stark focus. Help may be needed to deal with guilt, depression and family discord. In this time of crisis there is the possibility of resolving old problems and finding reconciliation that greatly strengthens the family (Saunders 1965).

Perhaps the discovery, and the telling, of truth also includes stopping the repression and hiding from each other about the hardships of the past. This sharing can be invaluable in understanding behaviour and healing hurts that may have not have had any personal connotation at all and where there was no realization of the effect it was having on others. Hurtful things, said and done, were misplaced attempts at expressing repressed nightmares.

After some resolution has been found, there is often an interesting shift in the music. The patient starts asking to hear the German folk music that he or she knew as a child. This was a part of life that had become taboo. Folk music melodies were usurped by the National Socialist propaganda machine and applied to other texts. This is still a problem in Germany as a whole cultural background of folk music has become tainted with Nationalist associations.

I have also worked with adult children who were ashamed of their parents and who had severed contact. They had returned because their parent was dying. Sitting in the room together and listening to the music at least allows them to be together peacefully and is often a decisive step to forgiveness and reconciliation. They can share in this therapeutic process and it is often a relief for them too (Kane *et al.* 1985).

Since I have transcribed much of this folk music for the Veeh Harp, I ask family members if they would like to play for their parents when it seems appropriate. (It is not necessary to read music to play this small harp.) Or their children have often asked me to accompany them so they can sing these old songs. This can bring the family together and a very tangible relaxation can be felt in the room when this happens. The patients' children tell me that this was an immense help in getting them to step over their own shadows and approach their parents. The hardness starts to melt and some of their emotional needs are being taken care of – letting the old negativity die and the good live on. Music can do this.

Sometimes patients will then want to prepare their funeral celebration that will reflect this healing process. Included in these preparations will be some of the music that we have used, prayers that have been said, some of their own words or those that have come to have special meaning. I often spend time with the family helping to pick out the music and arranging the musicians who will play.

Music during the process of dying

There are times when I play during the actual passing-on and I consider this to be a great privilege. Sometimes we are alone and sometimes the family is there. No matter what is happening on the 'other side', I feel strongly that the dying person should feel our love here. Music is surely well suited for this. It is a very personal way for me to say goodbye.

Coda

My life has changed as a result of this work. Without waxing too sentimental, the music has made it easier for me to open my heart. I have found a capacity to love that I did not know I had and an increased awareness of what it means to play music with love. It has made me aware of the importance of tolerance and of being mindful of the difference between sympathy and compassion. Sympathy saying, 'Oh you poor thing. Isn't that awful' and compassion announcing, 'I understand. I am here with you. Perhaps we can find a way to change something'.

I would like to quote from His Holiness the XIV Dalai Lama from a message he sent to a conference on 'Death, Dying and Living', held in Munich in 1996:

> The growth of interest in helping people die in peace with dignity is very encouraging. There is no greater way of repaying the kindness that each and every one of us has received at different stages of our lives than to offer help and comfort to those who are no longer able to help themselves. I offer my prayers that as we come to appreciate the importance of dying in peace, we will also begin to learn the key is to live in peace with ourselves and with others. (Dalai Lama 1996)

The Johannes Hospiz der Barmherzigen Brüder is a 25-bed facility in Munich, Germany, established in 1991. In 1998, the hospice admitted 438 patients, 225 females and 213 males, the average age being 68. In 1998, 314 patients passed on and 124 were released (returning home to die or going on to nursing homes); 392 were cancer patients, 3 HIV and 43 had other diseases. The average stay was 15 days.

CHAPTER 10

Working with Images and Recollection with Elderly Patients

Concetta M. Tomaino

The old person loses memory, which as a rule is the first faculty to be lost. Yet the old person has something poetic about him; in the popular mind he is prophetic, inspired. But recollection is indeed his best power, his consolation, which consoles him with its poetic farsightedness. (Kierkegaard 1845/1988)

Who we are as individuals is so linked to our memories and recollections of the past that it is difficult to imagine the loss experienced by those with dementia. Because the extent of this loss is often difficult to discern by standardized neuropsychological testing, one cannot predict the depth of awareness that remains in these individuals. Since 1978 I have had the privilege to work as a music therapist with many individuals diagnosed as having dementia. It is always remarkable to watch a person completely removed from the 'present' due to a disease such as Alzheimer's, a disease affecting nerve cells and neurotransmitters in the brain, come to life when a familiar song is played. The person's response may vary from a change in posture to animated movement: from a sound to verbal response. But usually there is a response, an interaction. Many times these seemingly disparate responses can reveal much about the preservation of self and the intact personal stories that may still remain.

Although much has been written on the use of music therapy with patients with dementia (Aldridge 1994, 1995; Bright 1972, 1981, 1988, 1991; Clair 1991; Gibbons 1977; Prickett 1988; Wheeler 1988), there are limited clinical data on the use of music of particular importance to an individual with dementia. I have observed, from my own clinical work, that songs of personal significance to a person with dementia can stimulate their responses. This has been indicated in the work of Gerdner and Swanson (1993) who suggested that the knowledge of the general category of musical interest may not be sufficient but rather knowledge of the specific type of music should be established prior to treatment.

This is indeed what I have discovered over the years. Music is not 'universal' with this population. Yes, certain melodies will soothe and others stimulate but to truly reach someone with dementia, on a personal level, his or her musical preferences must be taken into account. Favourite songs or pieces of music tend to receive more attention over one's lifetime and become ingrained in our memory. Over time, particular songs may come to represent significant events in one's life. Although attempts to investigate some aspect of these phenomena have been made (Prickett and Moore 1991; Wylie 1990), the effects of using songs of personal importance to persons with dementia within music therapy are not addressed in the literature. What is most remarkable is the extent to which music can play a significant role in allowing for the stories and recollections of persons with dementia to persist (Tomaino 1999). It is through the music that information can be presented and received within the music therapy sessions.

There is also a positive indication that familiar music can stimulate memory and improve reminiscence abilities in those with poor cognitive function (Sambandham and Schirm 1995; Tomaino 1996). One could argue that other forms of sensory stimulation, such as familiar photos and certain aromas, can trigger memory and reminiscence equally, yet the literature still shows that music has the strongest impact in persons with severe dementia when compared to other stimuli (Lord and Garner 1993; G. Smith 1986; Tomaino 1996).

The specifics of how music affects memory is still unknown, yet we feel the effects of music and memory every time we hear a favourite song. Music is capable of arousing deep and significant emotion in those who interact with it. John Sloboda (1989) described the autobiographical memories of musical events and the clarity of recall for adults who were asked to reminisce about early experience with music. Not only did they recall the musical event but also their physical reactions to the music were recalled as well. All memories were of events prior to the age of 10. Regardless of the number of years that had passed, the total memory of their early experience with music was still preserved. Does this hold true for personal events where music is just a component? Does listening to one's wedding song, for example, evoke the complete memory and feeling of that day?

Music is often so well preserved in our memories that only a fragment of a melody is needed to stimulate recall of the title or lyrics (Bartlett and Snelus 1980). Although a sound, such as a bell, can evoke a simple attention response, music reflective of an individual's past, for example songs of childhood, homeland or key life events, result in emotional reactions. It is the connections of the auditory nerve to key limbic structures in the brain that account for such emotionally charged responses to familiar music (Tomaino 1993b). The limbic area of the mid-brain has been indicated in long-term memory storage and emotional processing. Because memories persist when they have some personal importance for the individual, and the processing of familiar music seems to bypass higher cortical structures, it is possible to reach the 'sense of self' that may still be preserved in persons with dementia through the use of meaningful songs.

Schachtel (1947) stated that memory as a function of the living personality can be understood only as a capacity for the organization and reconstruction of past experiences and impressions in the services of present needs, fears and interests. Just as there is no such thing as impersonal perception and impersonal experience, there is also no impersonal memory. For this reason familiar songs may serve as a retrieval cue for memory recall. Rudy and Sutherland (1994), in discussing assumptions about theories of associative memory, stated that:

> a target memory is activated by retrieval cues whose representations are connected with the target memory in the network. The retrieval cues themselves are viewed as a set of independent environmental stimuli or as elements each having some representation in the network. The critical assumptions we then make are about how these cues cooperate or combine to retrieve a target memory. (Rudy and Sutherland 1994, p.121)

The concept of retrieval cues and memory is not new and, in fact, was first suggested by Richard Semon (1921), who argued that any given memory could be elicited by just a few select cues, the parts of the original experience that a person focused on at the time the experience occurred (Schacter 1996, p.58). A song can represent a gestalt of a period of one's life allowing for remembrance upon each listening of the familiar tune. Radocy and Boyle (1979) stated that:

> Listening to music of one's childhood or adolescence evokes feelings of childhood and adolescent experiences associated with the music...The power of music to elicit strong feelings of experiences associated with it provides individuals with a mechanism for re-experiencing many significant events within their lives. (Radocy and Boyle 1979, p.189)

Individuals with dementia have often lost the capacity to process many types of information. Even though the ability to identify a song may be gone, one can still respond emotionally to it. The response is almost spontaneous with no thought given to recognition of the song.

> These imagings, whether conscious or unconscious, are the stimuli to which the affective response is made. In short, music may give rise to images and trains of thought which, because of their relation to the inner life of the particular individual, may eventually culminate in affect. (Meyer 1956, p.256)

In addition to emotions, associations are also connected to musical memory and experience.

> It is the inner life of music which can still make contact with their inner lives, with them; which can awaken the hidden, seemingly extinguished soul; and evoke a wholly personal response of memory, associations, feelings, images, a return of thought and sensibility, an answering identity. (Sacks 1999, pp.11–12)

Other elements of music can also serve as retrieval cues. Dowling and Harwood (1986) explored the features of pitch and rhythmic organization that tend to make patterns difficult or easy to perceive and remember. They indicated that a listener's knowledge of a piece of music is stored in semantic memory and is integrated with other types of memory. The processing of the music takes place at both the conscious and subconscious levels. Research indicates that familiar elements of a song can trigger memory responses and associations. One aspect of a musical piece, be it melody, rhythm or lyrics, can trigger recall of each of the other components. If this is the case for those with normal mental functioning, how much does this hold true for those with cortical damage such as Alzheimer's? Such phenomena are evident clinically when a simple tapping of the melodic rhythm of a song can evoke recognition of the melody. Similarly, playing the first line of a song can cue recognition of the lyrics or song title. Swartz *et al.* (1992) suggested that individuals with Alzheimer's disease are capable of attending to and discriminating differences in fundamental music elements. In an earlier study they suggested that there is an independent neurological process for music processing as compared with language processing (Swartz *et al.* 1989).

Recall is thought to involve the search and retrieval of information in the memory store, whereas recognition is thought not to involve retrieval (Botwinick 1978, p.359). For the older person it is the telling of life stories over time that keep the memory alive. In the same sense, songs that one enjoys are listened to and sung over and over throughout one's life. This may help keep memories for songs stronger than other memories that may not be called to attention as often (Tomaino 1993a).

Observing people with dementia respond to music over these years has convinced me that there must be underlying neurological processes that enable them to respond so well to music when all else has failed, yet nothing that I read can explain why. The brain does not function like a homologous – each aspect of human function being assigned to a particular region of the brain – but, rather, as a dynamic, ever-changing system of interconnecting neurons that work in consort to produce our complex, dynamic, insights of and responses to the world around us. This is the concept of neural networks that has almost replaced the concept of localized brain function. The more I learn about these networks the more I wonder about the 'music connection' because so many skills are better preserved when music is a component of the learning process.

When I investigate music and memory, my definition of memory is very broad. Unlike a newborn child whose every experience is one of discovery, an adult's language, habits, and social skills are all based on information learned throughout the person's life. It is the comparison, both conscious and unconscious, of these verbal and affectual responses to previous life experiences, that I define as memory. New experiences are spontaneously compared to some similar event or set of responses in our long-term memory. Learning is an act of remembering; remembering an act of learning anew.

To study the potential of using preferred music to stimulate images and reminiscence in persons with dementia, I conducted a study with several women (Tomaino 1999). In each music therapy session I used songs that had been identified by each woman's family as being significant. Each session was videotaped and transcribed. The complete transcriptions, which included verbal as well as descriptive information, amounted to over 600 pages. As I read each page and analysed the content, I discovered that what I had originally thought to be meaningless jargon was indeed fragments of images and memories of these individuals. Independently, these phrases seemed to be unrelated or distantly related to what had taken place in the moment. Pieced together the phrases provided a congruent whole and a glimpse into the thoughts of these four women. The following short case histories introduce the four female participants and illustrate the images and recollections revealed during the sessions.

Molly

Molly was a quiet, soft-spoken 87-year-old woman who was born in Ireland and moved to London as a young woman. There is no record of when she arrived in the United States. She was admitted to our facility just two weeks before I began working with her.

Her son reported that his mother had been becoming progressively confused. She had fallen at home, hit her head, and was admitted to the local medical centre where she was found to have severe dementia. She was recommended for long-term placement. Her son was saddened by his mother's need for continued care but felt that our facility would provide the best care for her.

Molly spent most of her time over the past several years with her family. She enjoyed television game shows and James Cagney movies. She required assistance in activities of daily living which meant she needed someone to bathe and dress her. Although she could physically do these tasks, Molly no longer remembered how to do them. Her orientation was also impaired due to her dementia. She was unable to recall anything about herself or her family. She could just tell me her name, Molly. This is important to note here because during the course of music therapy she did provide information about her family. Molly was quiet during the music therapy sessions. Her facial expressions and spontaneous physical responses demonstrated to me from the first session that Molly was aware and responsive to me and the music. The feelings and emotions she demonstrated provided a glimpse of who Molly once was. I found her to be a loving, nurturing woman, who had become fearful as a result of her lack of understanding of the unfamiliar surroundings.

When I interviewed her son regarding Molly's favourite songs, he suggested Irish songs like 'When Irish Eyes are Smiling'. The songs I used in the first session were: 'When Irish Eyes are Smiling', 'Molly Malone', 'Donegal', 'Yankee Doodle Dandy', 'Over There', 'It's a Long Way to Tipperary', 'Let Me Call You Sweetheart', 'Irish Washerwoman', 'Immaculate

Mary' and 'London Bridge'. These songs were chosen as they reflected her personal identity and interests – being from Ireland and England, her Catholic religion (Immaculate Mary) and James Cagney (Yankee Doodle Dandy). Although I came back to these songs during the subsequent sessions, I also introduced other songs that were from the same musical genre and time period. In the second session and in subsequent sessions, I introduced new songs, which were similar, in an effort to engage Molly further in the music and in interactions with me.

I initially relied on these responses to determine which music to use in the subsequent sessions. For example, in my journal for Molly's first session, I noted that she was more responsive to the Irish songs than to some of the Irving Berlin tunes. I played both types of songs on the accordion and the songs were similar in rhythm. If this were just a spontaneous response to rhythm, without recognition or preference, she should have responded the same for both types of music, yet she consistently moved, smiled and attempted to sing more often with the Irish songs.

During the first session, after I played 'It's a Long Way to Tipperary' Molly started to cry. Later in the same session, after the song 'London Bridge', Molly tried to get out of her wheelchair. I asked if she was all right and she took my hand and kissed it and stated 'My mother's home, (mumbles) the kids are there'. Because Molly was often silent, these fleeting remarks, appearing spontaneously after particular songs and not others, caused me to examine if there was a relationship between a song of 'personal importance' and these 'thought fragments'. Indeed, in the fourth session, I observed her to be more attentive during 'It's a Long Way to Tipperary'. Although I played the song in the preceding sessions, this was the first time Molly sang some of the lyrics. Because she was so responsive and maintained eye contact with me, I continued to play another verse to keep her engaged. At the end she commented 'That's nice'. This was the most coherent and connected that Molly had been in a session. I took this opportunity to ask her some questions about herself.

C: Molly, where are you from?

M: Me? From Dublin? (Her hospital records had stated that she was from England so I asked her)

C: From England?

M: (She looks at me 'Oh England' and mumbles a few words.)

C: (I realized that she sincerely meant Ireland so I asked) From Ireland?

M:　　I was born there.

C:　　Where was everyone born?

M:　　County Cork.

C:　　Do you know where Dublin is?

M:　　Oh, easy to get to – nice little town.

C:　　Ever go to County Cork?

M:　　Beautiful.

Prior to this session Molly was able to tell me only her name. She could not answer any questions about her past. Yet in this session we were fully engaged in a meaningful exchange about her birthplace. The song connected her to a thought and she was able to maintain it for a short while. After the session, I spoke to Molly's son about her place of birth. He said that she was born in Ireland although she moved to England as a young child.

In our seventh session, shortly after the session began, I played 'An Irish Lullaby' and Molly looked sad. I then played the song, 'Does Your Mother Come from Ireland' after which Molly stated '54' then 'gotta have'. I played two other songs and Molly stated 'the key' and later on 'I want to go home'. Each word came after a song. I do not believe the songs interrupted her thoughts but rather helped her hold on to them.

In many instances recall did occur and was seemingly triggered by a particular song, or happened spontaneously within the session. In one session, when Molly mentioned her son's name I played the song 'O Danny Boy'. Although this was not her son's name, the song conveyed the idea of love for one's son. At the end of the song she sang the last line and then placed her hand on her chest. After the same song, several sessions later, she not only mentioned her son's name but also stated that she had not seen him for a while. She then asked if I had seen him. Considering that she was unable to relay any information about herself in the first session, this demonstrated change in memory was remarkable to me. It is also possible that our speaking about her son in the earlier session had been paired with the song. Then in the later session this pairing came back to her mind when she heard the song again. Because her short-term memory was so poor, I doubt if this were the case; however, the possibility is fascinating.

Sadie

Sadie was a 75-year-old woman who was born in Poland in 1918. Her family left Poland for Palestine, Israel, when Sadie was approximately 3 years old. She was one of four siblings and had one brother still living in Israel. Sadie received the equivalent of a high school education and completed seminary training there. She taught for a while and then came to the United States in 1949 to get medical treatment when she lost an eye in an accident. She married a family member of a successful company in 1951. They had one son and she returned to work when the boy was 14. She taught arts and crafts in a senior centre for a while. After her husband's death in 1988, her own health started to deteriorate.

Though the youngest of the participants, she looked old and frail. Her old photographs depicted her as a young elegant woman. The years and her illness had taken much away. She had been admitted to a local medical centre after a hip fracture and was found to have severe protein and caloric malnutrition. She was first admitted to our restorative rehabilitation programme at the son's request, but due to her confusion, was soon placed on one of the dementia units. Sadie presented herself as an anxious woman who was obviously fixated on her broken teeth. Sadie's son could provide only general categories of music but because Sadie was verbal, I hoped that she could tell me which of the songs were meaningful to her. The music used was a mixture of Israeli, Hebrew and Yiddish songs, as well as some Polish songs and some waltzes. I found that the music took her attention off her teeth and other problems as she would listen quietly as the music played but, as soon as the music stopped, continued voicing her worries.

In the first session I introduced: 'Tum Balalaika', 'Shein vi di L' vone', 'Pappirossen', 'Sholom A'leychem', 'Hussen Challa Mazeltov', 'Tzena Tzena', 'Merry Widow Waltz', 'Bashana Habaha' and 'O say Shalom'. I tried to introduce a different song in each session because I did not have much background information on her specific musical interests. During our first session Sadie was able to tell me that she lived in Manhattan but not much else. In subsequent sessions, especially after Israeli and Hebrew folksongs, she began speaking about being a teacher: 'I was an arts and crafts teacher'. With each session there were fragments of ideas and memories that were interspersed with her preoccupation about her current illness. I knew that she had taught at a New York senior centre but there was no record of her being a teacher in Israel, yet this was the image that persisted. Toward the last session, following the song 'Jerusalem of Gold' she remarked: 'I was a very good arts and crafts teacher…yeah, and now I lost everything'. With Sadie the awareness of loss was very great. The music helped to provide some comfort in the past, of a time and place when she was active and beautiful. It also made her conscious that things had changed although she was not sure what was different or how she had changed. In the last session she asked: 'What happened to me anyway?' I told her that she had been sick, to which she replied: 'No, I was sick?…I was a beautiful girl. Right? Beautiful, really. I don't know what I want to do…Sadila. [I ask her who called her Sadila] They used to call me Sadila'. As we continued to work together and her medical needs were taken care of, Sadie became more engaged in daily activities. Her comfort level continued to increase and the songs continued to serve as a bridge to memories that sustained her sense of comfort and security.

Rose

Rose was an 80-year-old woman with a pre-admission diagnosis of dementia, anemia, arteriosclerotic heart disease (ASHD), osteoporosis and pneumonia. She was born, in upstate New York, into a family with three brothers, all of whom were deceased. She most likely went to high school and then worked for her brother until he sold his business. Rose worked for a prominent newspaper as an ad taker until her retirement at age 65. She married in 1946 and her husband died only five years later at the age of 40 from rheumatic heart disease. She never remarried and the couple had no children. Her only significant other was her sister-in-law with whom she had been friends from before her marriage. They lived in the same building until recently. Rose enjoyed reading newspapers and magazines, going to movies, taking cruises and vacationing in the Catskills.

You could tell that Rose was a very social woman. She was friendly to everyone she met and the staff were already becoming friendly with her only days after her admission. She was very easy to get along with. Despite her apparent orientation to self and excellent verbal skills, she had shown no awareness of her new environment or that there was anything wrong with her.

Rose was placed on a unit that I was assigned to prior to the start of this study. I had the chance to work with her twice in the music therapy group I led on her unit. She liked to play a large tom-tom and would play the rhythm 'shave and a hair cut' which I would repeat on the accordion and then she would laugh. I knew from her reactions that she knew the song 'I Don't

Know Why I Love You Like I Do' and this became a key song in our sessions together. Her sister-in-law mentioned that Rose liked Frank Sinatra and most popular music of the late 1930s and early 1940s. I found from the admitting social worker, who got the information from Rose's sister-in-law, that Rose had many friends including male friends with whom she would socialize.

The songs I used during the sessions included songs from a tape of Frank Sinatra, for example 'I Remember Tommy', 'I'll be Seeing You' and 'Without a Song'. Additional songs such as 'There Goes my Heart' I played on the accordion or the piano.

For Rose, the sessions evolved around sitting at the piano with me and trying to play some of her favourite songs. Her memory from session to session improved as well. She remembered the songs that we played and especially the piano. In one session after I played 'I Don't Know Why', I asked her if she ever played the piano. She replied: 'Yeah I did but at that time it wasn't such a big, such a big, ah you know...but I don't think I have it now any more'. After a few more songs she continued her thought: 'A long time ago, you know, before I went to work, you know, and ah, you know, we had a piano'.

Her memory of the piano and the studio carried over from session to session. She talked about playing the piano when she was smaller. 'I had a piano like that, one time'. I asked her where it was and she said: 'In the living room'. She then said that she would have to look at it when she got back because she forgot what it looked like. 'I think I always had it in my house, no my mother's house'. I asked her where was her mother's house and she replied: 'It was like a park or something'. She remembered that she played it but could recall only a few memories of the piano. 'I know I have the same kind of colour but I when I get home'. I asked who else played the piano and she said she thought that she was the only one.

R: And I had this other one, and I don't know what happened to it now.

C: Well your sister Elsie said that it was at your mother's house.

R: I don't think so. Well in the first place she wouldn't know what to do with it. It was in this place and she doesn't have a piano, and uh, I didn't have it either but uh I got used to it but uh I didn't really have all these. Sometimes I do it right away, and sometimes I didn't know to do it.

Rose started to remember other information about herself as our sessions together progressed, though at times she forgot that she had just seen me on her unit the same morning. She also started to remember that she was not at home and that she had changed. 'Sometimes I get lonely…Yeah, because I was the only girl in the house and ah sometimes you had to go out you'd to go out to work or someplace like that and I stay in then and then I stopped doing that little things that I, I remember [looks more serious]'. I asked her what kinds of things she did when she was home. 'At home I don't hardly do anything, on it, nothing really, unless they call me on the phone or something and want to say something and that's about it. But also maybe I, um, I'm working'. She also began to remember my name. 'Connie when I was coming from the hospital I…think I know this one – [points to my ID]'. 'I wasn't too sure about the name…Now I am, and ah, I was thinking about you, you know? For some reason you weren't here, and I was thinking, I wonder where is Connie'.

Rose continued to recall bits and pieces of the preceding sessions and of other activities in her life. She became confused, however, when she tried to integrate the past images and memories, that would spontaneously come to her, with the reality of her present condition and placement at the nursing home. This did not seem to frustrate her, but it did confuse her at times. Her memory of playing the piano became an integral part of our sessions. It was interesting for me to learn that she had a piano in her mother's house only when she was very young. Yet her images of the piano were still very vivid. In the final session Rose told me of how she was now playing the piano and everyone seemed to like it (she could play only single random notes, but the staff gave her a lot of encouragement). Her childhood memory of the piano, and whatever associations that brought to her, were still richly connected to the present and somehow became her reality in 'playing' the piano every day.

Carmen

Carmen was the oldest of the participants but she definitely did not look her 87 years. She was born in Puerto Rico and lived in an orphanage until she was adopted by an American family and brought to the United States at the age of 2. She finished high school and worked briefly until her marriage to John. They had one son whom they named John. Her husband took her back to Puerto Rico where she met her blood relatives for the first time. She remained in Puerto Rico for six years, causing her husband to leave her. She remarried after meeting her second husband where they worked. He had some problems that caused the couple to separate. She remained close to her son, 'the love of her life'.

She used to enjoy sewing and listening to music. Her son was very involved and visited Carmen almost every evening. He said that she loved to sing especially popular Latin songs. She also enjoyed songs sung by Frank Sinatra and Tony Bennett.

The music I used included a recording of Eydie Gorme singing some Latin tunes and the Frank Sinatra tape that I used for Rose. In the first sessions I included a recording, primarily mambos, of Tito Puente which I thought Carmen might know since she enjoyed Latin dance music. She did not convey any interest in or familiarity with the music so I did not use the tape in the rest of the sessions. I used many of the Latin songs with Carmen as a stimulus for conversations about her son or her family, her two favourite topics. At other times, though, her recollections were more obscure. In one session, for example, she tried to tell me something about her son. She was unable to think of what it was so I played a song, 'Besame Mucho', which she had told me was her son's favourite song. She interrupted the song and stated that she wanted to hear something Jewish. She then started to talk about her son. When I asked her where he worked she said:

Ca: In New York where I work, here in a store.

C: In a store?

Ca: Not in a store, but you know where I was. I always had three chairs sitting there for for for putting the buildings the bellies on them, and the, with all of those things on them you know, you know, you know.

C: What kind of work did you do?

Ca: Ay, ay...I still had, ah, to work when he came in.

C: You had to work?

Ca: No, I took over the tips for...the chicks standing over for beer, was there you know, for instance, you have sitting along...He was always right, really. Take it and then have four children... all this talk about John and this gives me it takes a picture it makes me ill. No for him. George Gomez.

C: Who's that?

Ca: I don't know I heard them out there from the street.

At other times after I played the songs 'DeColores', 'Guantanamera' or 'Celito Lindo', Carmen mentioned something about Christmas. In one session she actually visualized a Christmas tree. After I finished playing the song there was a long pause and then Carmen pointed to the wall.

Ca: The Christmas tree.

C: Where?

Ca: Where? In the Center.

C: Is it decorated?

Ca: No.

In a later session after I play 'Guantanamera', Carmen stares at me and asks:

Ca: Where did my father go?

C: I don't know. Carmen, you look tired, I am going to take you back soon.

Ca: I am hungry. CHRISTMAS!

C: Christmas?

Ca: Yeah, are you hungry for Christmas?

Looking back over my notes and video of the sessions, I realized that Carmen mentioned Christmas several times. In every instance, Carmen looked deep in thought, almost transfixed, after listening quietly to these songs. Because the sessions took place during the summer months there were no environmental elements to stimulate her recollections of Christmas time, yet this was the consistent image that kept returning to her.

Conclusion

Human memory is complex and goes deeper than that which is visibly tangible. What I have found fascinating in each of the women mentioned above, and indeed in many of the individuals with whom I have worked, is that music can stimulate images and recollections where mere words and photos cannot. Somehow, somewhere, there is a link to preserved function if the right set of circumstances or the right stimulation is provided. I believe that it is the pairing of music to significant events that strengthens its use as a retrieval cue. There is also a possibility that this pairing results in the activation of a different neural network or recruits different neurological systems that allow for the retrieval of images and recollections. Although areas of convergence and various neural networks have been discussed in the literature (Damasio 1994; Rose 1992), the underlying processes of music stimulated recall need further investigation. Nevertheless, clinical study indicates that familiar music can be a powerful stimulus. A song can be an engram, a code, a representation of a piece of one's history. In the particular women described above, I observed intact personalities and images that continued to unfold during the course of the music therapy sessions despite the severe cognitive deficits these women presented in all areas of function. All of the songs I used repeatedly in the sessions represented something to each of the women. Familiar music did serve as a catalyst to disclose past associations. Molly's connection to Ireland, Sadie's connection to Israel, and Rose's memory of the piano in her mother's living room all demonstrated that the music was needed to access these associations. As I gained an understanding of each woman's response to certain songs, I then purposefully chose a song to stimulate, reflect and/or support her verbalizations. For example, I consciously chose a song such as 'Oh Danny Boy' to connect to Molly when she mentioned her son. What I discovered is that many seemingly lost memories still exist and can be stimulated with familiar music. The stream of consciousness, the random words, the visual images all were presented at the end of a song. As the sessions progressed, some of these thoughts became more coherent. I could not anticipate the responses or outcomes I received as one can never predict how a person with dementia will respond at any given time. It is only in the process of careful observation and analysis of each individual's response to various music that such understanding occurs.

Songs referred to in the chapter

Many songs were used in the therapy sessions described. The following are the references for those particular songs cited in this chapter.

Songs for Molly

Molly Malone: traditional Irish, 1978 Robbins Music Corp.

When Irish Eyes are Smiling: words by Chauncey Olcott and Geo. Graff Jr, music by Ernest R. Ball, 1912 M. Whitmark and Sons renewed by Chappell and Co. Inc.

Yankee Doodle Boy: words and music by G.M. Cohen, 1948 Jewel Music Publishing Co. Inc. and Harrison, Music Corp. New York.

It's a Long Way to Tipperary: words and music by Jack Judge and Harry Williams by B. Feldman and Co. London. Renewed by Chappell and Co. Inc.

Let Me Call You Sweetheart: words by Beth Slater Whitson, music by Leo Frieman, 1910 Shawnee Press Inc.

Irish Washerwoman: traditional Irish, 1981 Hal Leonard Publishing Co.

Immaculate Mary: Lourdes hymn by Jeremiah Cummings, 1814–66 Grenoble 1882.

London Bridge: traditional English.

Did Your Mother Come from Ireland: words and music by Jimmy Kennedy and Michael Carp, 1936 World Copyrights ltd, renewed Chappell and Co. Inc.

Danny Boy: Adapted from Old Irish Air by Fred E. Weatherly, words by same.

Over There: words and music by G.M. Cohen, 1917 renewed 1945 Leo Feist Inc.

Songs for Sadie

Tum Balalaika: A. Bitter, 1940.

Shein vi di Lívone: music by Joseph Rumshinsky, words by Chaim Tauber, 1938 Henry Lefkowitch, New York.

Pappirossen: words and music by H. Yablokoff, 1956 J. and J. Kammen Music Co., New York.

Sholom Aíleychem: I. and S.E. Goldfarb, 1954 Accordion Music Publishing Co., New York.

Hussen Challa Mazeltov: traditional Hebrew.

Tzena: words by Issachar Miron (Michrovsky).

Merry Widow Waltz: Franz Lehar.

Bashana Habaha: traditional Hebrew.

O say Shalom: traditional Hebrew.

Jerusalem of Gold: Yerushaláim shel zahav – words and music by Naomi Shemer 1967 Assigned to Chappell and Co., London.

Songs for Rose

I'll Be Seeing You: words and music by Irving Kahal and Sammy Fain, 1938 by Williamson Music Inc. Administered by Chappell and Co.

Without a Song: words by William Rose and Edward Eliscu, music by Vincent Youmans.

I Don't Know Why I Love You Like I Do: words by Roy Turk, music by Fred E. Ahlert, 1931 and renewed 1959 Cromwell Music Inc., New York.

There Goes My Heart: words by Benny Davis, music by Burt F. Bacharach, 1964 by Anne-Rachel Music Corp. Blue Seas Music Inc. and Jac Music and Co. All rights administered by Chappell and Co.

Songs for Carmen

DeColores: Spanish folk.

Cilito Lindo: Spanish folk, 1923 EMI Miller Catalog Inc.

Besame Mucho: words and music by Consuelo Velazquez, 1941 by Promotora Hispano Americana de Musica.

You Belong To My Heart: words and music by Agustin Lara,1941 Promotora Hispana Americana di Muscia, English lyrics by Ray Gilbert.

Guantanamero: Spanish folk, 1963 Fall River Music Inc.

Mas Amor: words and music by Steve Lawrence and Eydie Gorme, Westside Music inc. BMI

Luna Lunara: Peer International Corp, BMI.

Desesperademente: Peer International Corp, BMI.

Roman Guitar: Alfred Music Co. Inc. ASCAP.

No Te Vayas Sin Mi: Edward B. Marks Music Corp. BMI.

Recordings

Naomi Shemer Sings Her Famous Jerusalem of Gold. Capitol Records DT 10510.

Michael Coleman/The McNulty Family – Irish Dance Party. Coral Records CRL 57464

Eydie Gorme More Amore Edyie Gorme and The Trio Los Panchos. Columbia CL2376

Cuatro Vidas –Four lives

No Te Vayas Sin Mi – Don't leave without me

Mas Amor – More love

Guitarra Romana – Roman guitar

Luna Lunera – Bright moon

Frank Sinatra – I Remember Tommy – Capitol Records

Tito Puente – the Mambo King: RMM Records and Video. RMFC – 80680.

CHAPTER 11

We'll Survive

An Experiential View of Dance Movement Therapy for People with Dementia

Marion Violets

For people with neural damage, bewildering and disturbing things happen frequently.

In the layout in several residential homes, where I often forget which floor I am on, or which direction I am going in, it is not surprising that there is an all-pervasive theme of being bewilderingly and sometimes angrily lost.

'Why can't I go home?' 'Where is everyone I love?' 'Why have I got nothing in my pocket?' 'I just can't seem to find my purse.' 'Where are those keys? You know the ones that, that…you know…that open…the thingy, the flat one, it's blue…'

This is the stuff of nightmare, where you are suddenly starring in your own horror movie.

For a therapist coming into this situation it is a priority to be a 'present' listener (Kitwood 1997). However bizarre the seeming content of the conversation, the fact that the person feels sad, frightened and bewildered by what is happening to them is only too real. Affirming their feeling gives validity to their experience and restores some sense of belonging and reality for both client and therapist.

I often experience the feeling that it is *me* who is in a strange land without a map or compass, not knowing the language and that it is up to me to learn the way from the people who are living there. I am frequently amazed and inspired by the intrinsic genius of people who have to survive and find a way to communicate when there are no longer terms of reference in common, especially verbally. Movement, music, song, dance and play offer another possibility of expressing the imaginative self and a whole wealth of information about a person, if only we can enter into this frame of reference.

Short-term memory and verbal and intellectual pathways are usually the first to disappear in the neural landscape. However, the 'body brain' remembers and longs for free expression. If we try to subdue this body memory in order to imitate what is often called 'appropriate behaviour' in western countries, we block the communication channels which are the life expression for people with neural damage. We are then cutting ourselves off from a whole world of exciting information that they can bring to us, as a creative contribution to living knowledge.

The resources that people with dementia can bring to us are offered so openly because of their congruent behaviour. This openness is often confusing to the rest of us who have learned to develop many devious strategies in order to survive the layers of social complexity and it is often easier and less threatening to dismiss their 'language' as 'difficult' or 'incomprehensible' behaviour (Stokes 1995).

When I began dance movement therapy with people with neural damage, I realized that the work that we had been doing in the field of creative therapies was now being given credence by neuroscientific research. What we had observed and understood in our experiential work was being proved in scientific terms. What we had witnessed, that changes in body movement behaviour could change the way a person thinks and feels, had been confirmed. Now an area of the brain had been located where it had been demonstrated that the energy for thought and movement was derived from the same source (Damasio 1994, 2000). Carla Hannaford (1995) also shows how damaged neural pathways might be re-routed. The practical orchestration of this has also been presented in the work of the innovative physiotherapist Sophie Levitt (1995) working with children with brain injury.

When I was asked to develop a movement programme for older people I felt that the basis for the method I was developing was on the right track.

I soon discovered that 'older people' covered a wide span of all types of people over an age range from 50 to 100+ describing those who were very fit and active, both mentally and physically, to those suffering with varying types and degrees of dementia, including Alzheimer's. Other people in this large category might be fragile through physical impairment, mental health problems, stroke damage or Parkinson's.

This was supported by an ongoing debate among clients themselves about all being lumped together as a category, when there is such a wide divergence of different needs, 'as though we are all the same because we are older'.

Background of the journey towards developing a model for this work

For many years I had been working with the moving circle as a form of integration and communication. I had worked with groups of adults and children in Britain, France, briefly in Bosnia during the war and also in Canada and the United States. I often used community and circle dances, both traditional and modern choreographies, as a means of bringing the group into a secure place, where people could communicate feelings and ideas to each other within a framework of exploration. The changes I witnessed in people as we worked, were so astonishing in many instances, that I became absorbed in trying to define exactly what it was that created the possibility for healing, often in severe cases of both mental and physical anguish. This had been particularly noticeable in traumatized children whose appearance changed dramatically within minutes of dancing with others in the circle. The disengaged eye focus came back into the present surroundings, the colour changed from grey pallor to a warm pink skin colour, the breathing pattern deepened and there was a sudden smile like someone waking out of a long sleep.

I looked at the components in the work. There was the dance. Many of the dances were very old and were based in ancient traditions of community. They united people in synchronistic rhythm to face issues of life and death, rooted in the organic pattern of the seasons. A common experience of joy and pain was all in here (Wosein 1986). The new choreographies were based very much on this concept. They linked the experience of body, mind and spirit to the rhythm of life and the universality of the process.

There was the music. This was also often based in ancient tradition and had cadences which took people into another level of awareness and communication. Often there were songs and chants which enabled the group to use their voices together to bring the rhythm for the universal movement and new compositions had been especially written to facilitate this level of awareness.

There was the form of the circle itself. The connection between the group, where everyone had an equally seen and felt place, was a fundamental part of this unity. The form developed as a tangible and also flexible structure. There was a container for members of the group to share and develop their own movements. This was a part of the 'warm up', which could be developed later in the session where the whole group could work together while they explored their own individual dance movements (Leventhal 1979). This part of the work could extend into a group choreography, sometimes with voice rhythm accompaniment.

There was the facilitator/therapist/teacher. The names sometimes varied because they could each apply, in different circumstances. It was evident that the presence and facilitation by this person, was a powerful ingredient in the healing process.

The process. In terms of quantum physics, it was not these items as intrinsic modalities but rather the relationship of the components to each other. The whole organism was involved in an interactive and participatory process, which created the dynamic for the functioning of the group. What I could see happening was that the moving communication was enabling the group to respond to each other physically and verbally more openly because they had taken the non-verbal route.

When I was asked to set up a movement and dance programme by a charity for brain injured children, the circle form was an obvious choice. I had started using a wide repertoire of not only dances but also song experience games which I had adapted and added to my repertoire from my work with Education through Music in Canada and the United States (Richards 1986). For children who were essentially non-verbal in their forms of communication, the music, movement and song rhythms created new channels through which to access relationship and cognitive development. The underlying base of creative repetition through rhythm and play was fundamental to the process. Once the children were secure in the familiarity of the structure, the circle could expand or contract. It could move out from a sitting chair form to a standing base and then open again to the wider space so that individual expression and group movement communication could be interactive (Leventhal 1980).

The nature of how the circle operated in this process became, for me, a focus of attention. In her work with children with autism, Tina Erfer (1993) had already written about the need for a safely bounded structure so that the young people could focus on the work of the group. In the development of the model I was using, the songs and repetition of the movement and words which included the names of the people in the group, seemed to build the safe base circle form as a physical object. It then developed an elasticity. I experienced the circle working as the transitional space that Winnicott

(1971) described as the essential, safely held container, within which children could explore and develop their relationship with others and the outer environment. In developmental terms, the prime carer would create this safe space. In this specific situation, it was the therapist who defined the boundaries. During the pilot scheme which we ran in a local secondary school, it became very clear that the young people were being able to rework their relationships and co-ordinate their learning with their activity in the outer environment, through the security of the circle group which physically expanded and contracted with them like a skin.

When I was asked to set up groups with older people with dementia, the link with neural damage was the key to developing the circle model I had been using. (The connection being the neural damage, not working with adults as though they were children.) The task was then to adapt the method so that it would be appropriate for this population. Although I also worked with clients one to one, I felt that interaction and relationship were the prime needs for this group of people so that they could enjoy a better quality of life. I felt that this could be best achieved by finding the support of relationship and communication with peers and others in group activity which could return a sense of cohesion and belonging to those who could easily feel abandoned and rejected by the main stream of society.

In settings where this had not happened before, there was often complete disbelief on the part of the staff, as to how people with such individualistic needs could be encouraged to hold their focus long enough to stay in a group at all. In other settings there was already a tradition of something called 'gentle exercise' which was based on a group working in a chair and wheel-chair circle. There were groups already operating in this way, using varying models including those within dance movement therapy. This was not usually understood by the setting and was (is) rarely paid for as therapy but rather as an exercise activity, often funded as classes or sessions by adult education, social services or the setting itself. Consequently it was often difficult to organize groups in a confidential, therapeutic environment. They usually had to be held in open spaces like dining rooms and be subjected to visitations from nursing staff taking clients in and out, visitors and others.

Still one of the most difficult parts of the process is to find support for physically bringing the group together from busy staff who are trying 'to get things done' and to whom this could seem like an unimportant activity. I frequently witness empathetic caring by the staff for their clients, although they themselves are often over-stretched and unsupported, certainly by any psychological supervision. I have often heard them express their fears that this might happen to their parents, if they are young, or themselves, as they become more mature. This fear is frequently the underlying theme behind the various defensive attitudes adopted by anyone who works in this kind of environment. These might surface in behaviour patterns of babying the client, being brisk and matter of fact and not having time to listen to what might be termed as 'incomprehensible ramblings', or teasing and joking, often of a sexually humorous nature. The fact that in a movement group, clients can become totally absorbed and stay focused for an hour, when they would normally not be able to concentrate for more than a few moments, is not usually lost on the discerning, even if they cannot explain it and find it mystifying.

What was recognizable as being important by the staff was the 'gentle exercise' and for this a seated circle was understood. The circle and group dynamic became a physical boundary. It created a therapeutic space even if the group had to be held in communal facilities (Keady and Nolan 1995).

Practical application of the model

Coming into this kind of setting I considered that the first priority was to engage clients who were separated and isolated in their own frame of reference, encouraging them to come into the group and connect with others. The initial work was to facilitate a safe base within which cohesiveness could develop. From my previous experience, I knew that I would have to use my own physical dynamic, through my voice and movement, for us to build the 'nascent' group (Sandel and Johnson 1983, 1987). I had to be a conductor for verbal communication, connecting each member of the group, through me, to each other, until the physical form of the circle group had established itself strongly enough for me to 'step back'.

I needed a technique to engage clients who often seemed out of reach. They were either very passive and abstracted or sleepy, anxious and restlessly moving, preoccupied with something very important which others were not able to translate and above all, existing, isolated in their own world. How could I interest and involve someone who moved in this kind of pattern, especially to bring them together as a group?

My main resource for the method of engagement is the use of balls of different textures and sizes. The person who might seem far away and says they cannot do anything, suddenly comes into the present when their body finds itself able to catch and throw the ball. Often the catching is a surprise and then the client wants to know what to do with it and to whom they might send it. This gives the opportunity to locate others in the group and to begin a web of connections. As the therapist I underline every action verbally, repeating how the person has caught the ball, which part of the body it has touched. I emphasize the quality and the relationship of the movement: is it strong, hard, soft or light? Exactly how each person connects by throwing or receiving the ball presents the group with revealing information. Under arm, over arm, or the ball may be carefully passed to the next group member; whether it is bounced across with difficulty or thrown up high can remind each person about the potential of their movement landscape and can link them to forgotten memories and thinking processes.

We also work with kicking the ball: in almost every case the feet seem to know immediately what to do, even in very frail clients who have severe stroke damage. As the movements become stronger and I underline more what each person is achieving, there is an increase in confidence and focus of interest, shown in the lifting of posture and alertness of gaze.

Working from the theory that certain kinds of neural damage cause difficulty in receiving abstract concepts and the knowledge that the body brain has its own memory pathways, I use the method of proprioceptive touch, that is giving a body prompt. Sometimes because of neural damage, clients might lose connections with certain body parts, such as not being able to connect that the feet or hands belong to the rest of their body. This is when I use a light touch prompt, attaching the word and movement description to the body part. This is far more effective if it can be consistent and repeated over time (Holden 1987).

This method may seem to be unusual compared to the more open expressive work normally associated with the creative therapies. What needs to be looked at here is that the apparent directive method is not didactic instruction, as in an educational model, but a creative repetition of a physical frame of reference which connects the individual's body with the containing framework. The subsequent map, designed between therapist and group, becomes the flexible structure upon which the group can build its independence.

It often feels like building up a three-dimensional model of an intricate landscape which requires patience and time and meticulous creative repetition. The body memory, which the ball prompts, locates the person with their own latency period of development, when the group or gang would be playing together, still held within the safety of the wider parental structure

but able to experiment with relationships within the group through movement and play. The work I had done with the Education through Music
programme reminded me of my own childhood knowledge and wonderful
storehouse of singing, circle movement games, often using a ball. (Probably
this can be regarded as a bonus of pre- and post-Second World War social
deprivation, where children were able to play safely, in groups together in
the street, without vehicles or other dangers. These rhyming, song and
movement games included a lot of innovation and regional variation.) For
older people who had grown up with this kind of play, the rhythm, song and
movement circle was very comfortable and familiar.

The fear of fragmentation and falling apart brought up attachment
anxieties without exception. Often clients would say 'I must let my mother
know where I am' or 'My mother would not like me doing that'. The circle
group provided the held space for this to be expressed and to find a base
which provided the familiar safety for the individual to act as their own
remembered self (Mahler, Pine and Bergman 1975). There was usually a time
when the controlling superego would pour scorn on the activity. The ability
to play and dance was often surrounded by fears that they would be seen to
be 'mad', a terror with which most clients were desperately struggling. In the
early sessions there would be a vacillation between these two states.

Assessments

This form of circle work has proved to be a very powerful and holding
container with a porous membrane-like skin. It is adaptable and protective. It
can stretch and shed, hold some things in and let others flow out. It can be
adjusted to fit the needs and growth of the group. From the contact with their
own movement repertoire and body language, the person with neural
damage is then able to translate information from their inner landscape of
feelings and thoughts so that they are able to innovate and discover ways to
communicate this to others within the circle.

This has to be repeated over and over again, maybe for many weeks, until
the group builds itself as an object of reference, where the members are
relating to each other and not just through the physical and emotional
presence of the therapist. It is from this moment, as the group moves into the
foreground, that the therapist can begin to recede towards the background.

Process of this development

We had found that we could spend longer and longer in just passing the ball. As the weeks progressed, the group had become absorbed in the dialogue which was able to develop. How all kinds of fears, attractions and experiments could be worked on through this method had allowed the game to become an enabling language. People had managed to develop sophisticated strategies, like pretending to throw and then throwing somewhere else. This had become an extended and fascinating game with much laughter and also an arena where underlying disputes and antagonisms could be worked out. As the therapist, my role had been to articulate the process and encourage others to reflect and consider the possibilities of what might be happening in the relationships. For the group, as their trust in the structure had grown, they had been able to risk sharing previously frightening and fragmenting thoughts; for example, not being liked, being overwhelmed with confusion and unable to do anything or feeling angry with someone else.

At first glance, the apparent openness of such a group as this could seem difficult to facilitate within therapeutic parameters. However, it appeared that the structure of the circle form, with its repetition of method and pattern of movement and song, could allow us the freedom to be creative within it. This meant not only that we could move more expressively but also that we could bring into the process events from the wider environment. The circle group acquired such a belief and strength in itself that it could encompass whatever happened.

Other parts of the structure

I found that the physical prop had such a specific role in enabling connection and focus that I also used stretch cloths, ropes and silk scarves. We worked with them in every session, which gave a confidence to people who then knew what was coming next. (In a landscape where perception can be changing and fragmenting from minute to minute, this kind of predictability is a very enabling focus.) What happened with these props was always different. This would depend on the exact composition of the group and issues presented. What might seem like 'the same old thing' to outsiders was endlessly intriguing to the group because of the infinite variability of the human psyche and the speed of perceptual change for this population. There was the richness of the creative imagination of people whose previously restrained and predictable pattern of language had now been released through dysphasia to a form of poetic expression. Often the unusual juxtaposition of words described a feeling so exactly, a poet laureate would die for it. For example the billowing cloth, as it became convex, was described as 'the sky ball-bowl'.

Some groups were able to develop physical skills of co-ordination which made the ball in the pond game a form of gymnastic agility, in which larger and larger movements could enable a count of tossing the ball in the cloth up to the ceiling fifty times, for example. (This group was originally composed of people who did not relate at all and who all said they had so many aches and pains they could not do anything. At the end there were often eighteen participants.) Other groups might work in a much more intricate way, intrigued by the way the ball could change direction by altering their style of movement. Often this would give the opportunity for tension lying below the surface to explode and to resolve. The physical form of the movement of the concave and convex cloth, matched the rise and fall of the anger and grief, excitement and lassitude.

The part of the session where we used special hand-painted silk scarves gave an opportunity for a different quality of movement and emotional expression. The fact that the scarves had been especially made for the work always brought the group into focus. They were able to value the colour and texture and to feel that it made them, as individuals, special also. I often put on gentle, lyrical music and encouraged people to make flowing movements which contrasted with the strong and often heavy weighted moves that they had been working with previously. I usually anchored this in practical use, showing how with a twisting movement we could open the chest area and lift the waist and ribs. I would actually make the contrasting movements myself, changing from a strong, deep-seated movement, to a light uplifted flowing gesture. This was very important in locating the clients spatially, so that they could develop their movement repertoire in this way. For most people, with the exception of one or two who had been used to dancing, this light flowing movement was unusual. In general, for the men in the group, it was often noted as not being 'manly'. Because the clients were so anxious about their identity, which was threatened by fragmentation, and because they felt that they were being watched for 'crazy' behaviour, they were often uneasy about trying anything which made them look 'peculiar'. Connecting the movements more to the practical aspects of the exercise increased their confidence. The joy and fluidity which they felt, once they had been able to experience them as a bodily sensation, increased their emotional satisfaction. They were then free to experiment further, in a more openly expressive style.

Development – music, song and dance – creative expression

One of the major difficulties for people with this kind of neural damage is the problem with spatial awareness and balance which causes lots of falls. Staying seated but finding ways of using the whole body and mind does give a safe base, while enabling the client to extend their imagination. From the part of the session where the group was using flowing movements with the scarves, we discovered the ability to move into a more freely expressive space. A dance could develop from how people could experiment with the movements made with the scarves, in relation to each other. An absorbing dialogue often developed between the group. People could innovate, mirror and reflect each other's movements. Reminiscence and singing often played a strong part in this. Sometimes people felt confident enough to stand with me and dance in the centre, while the others sang. Sometimes a few were able to hold each other for support, in synchronous movements of a circle dance. Because all this was able to take place within the holding circle, everyone was included whether they were able to stand or not. Often the one who remembered the words of the song was put in the minstrel role; others who were able to tell even fragments of stories, prompted by the movement and activity, were able to bring the whole group into shared memories. In this space they were able to feel and relate to their own identity as a valued member of a group, each with an important part to play. The familiar song lines connected a whole group in collectively remembered identity, when verbal patterns had already fragmented individuals into isolated chaos.

I found that this kind of development took place in a group at about the twelfth session and from there, this level of exchange accelerated. There was, by then, such a strong and flexible base for communication, it was possible for a range of psychotherapeutic issues to be addressed. By this stage, the instillation of hope, universality of the situation and cohesion of the group, all essential ingredients in the therapeutic process, were strongly present (Yalom 1995).

Case studies

The outsider

It became very clear that when someone was being 'wild', either shouting or withdrawing, it always empowered that person if their communication could be translated. So-called 'difficult behaviour' was invariably a desperate plea for communication, a cry of anguish from the continuously misunderstood. I found that if I could imagine what I would be trying to say, were I to find myself in this extreme situation of loss of liberty and identity, my communicative skills would be considerably sharpened. It was important for me, if I could, to articulate clearly the angry and upset feelings that were impossible to articulate in a verbal form recognizable to others, by someone under this kind of stress.

This would often happen to someone outside the group. They might be feeling disturbed and abandoned by this close-knit community, who might seem oblivious of their pain and isolation.

For example, Kevin would sometimes come shouting and very angry into the room where our quite large group was having noisy fun. If I asked him what was making him angry and repeated to the group that Kevin was angry and what did they think was upsetting him, he would be able to make it clear what he wanted to express. He never would join the group but always kept watch on the main door so that visitors could be let in. He would get very angry if we were so preoccupied that we did not hear the door. Recognizing him as the doorkeeper and the news-bringer was an important contact between him and the group. The shouting changed and he took his role as the link between the outer world and us. He would sit outside the group, near the door; once his role had been secured, he would sometimes join in the songs and even add others from his own repertoire, which could sometimes give us an innovative line for development.

Reality and paranoia

Sometimes people in this situation become aggressive or suffer paranoid delusions, when they feel they are no longer free. The fact that they are no longer free is real; the form of the delusions vary.

One dramatic but not extraordinary event was when Maeve came into the room where the circle had assembled, preparing for the movement group. She stopped and declaimed with outstretched arms, calling out: 'You fools, can't you see we're all prisoners here?'

People looked either mildly uneasy or accepting because she 'was ill'. My personal feelings were that we were in a truly dramatic reality in which the participant had said exactly what was terrifyingly true. It was the rest of us who were in denial.

Maeve desperately wanted to go home. She could remember the road name, which was not far away, but her family could not cope with her at home and there was no question of her being able to return there, so her statement was one of fact. From this point her imagination, and her fears of abandonment, embroidered an elaborate plot in which most of us featured. This included other kindly and innocent residents who were often accused of being in league with 'them' and who were passing the messages through their sticks to 'them down below' as they passed by her.

Mostly I was called to her rescue and pleaded with, to assist in her escape. I was seen as 'good' because the one place she found herself and felt safe was in the circle of the movement group and then 'as bad as the rest' when I would not let her out of the door. If she could be encouraged to come into the circle, it was here that her fragile, haunted ghost, which usually wandered round and round the corridors looking for the way out, became free and full of fun. Suddenly she remembered how to co-ordinate her movements, to throw the ball and to laugh and joke with the others as her friends and also to express her anxieties and dislikes. The transformation between the two was instant and truly astonishing. This was a clear example of how the 'safe base' worked.

Relationships

The friends

At first when I introduced myself and suggested that the two friends might like to join the group, they were very suspicious. 'We're all right here,' they said, 'we're together'. Once the circle of chairs had been formed in the large light dining room of the residential home, they found themselves in it somehow. Neither of them could resist the ball and both were very able and co-ordinated with it. Although Holly continued to denigrate it by saying that it was silly, child's stuff, she soon realized the skill involved and warmed to the praise. For her, the anxiety that people might think she was a bit 'gone in the head' often increased her panic and disorientation. We worked on this in the group, relating the skilfulness of the tasks we were performing with the building of interaction and support within the group.

Often Vera would be the one to encourage her friend and the others by saying that she did not care about what anyone said, because that was their problem and they were missing all the fun. She developed her own confidence over the weeks from the increase in her own co-ordination skills and her ability to survive what she had previously felt to be insurmountable difficulties. When she first came into the group she was over protective of Holly, saying that she (Holly) could not do things, because she was not well. She also extended this statement to herself and was often angry when someone threw the ball and it came at her too hard. Sometimes, if a conflict was brewing through issues that had been going on outside the group, a badly aimed ball which might hit her on the nose, for example, would be taken very personally, especially if this had been thrown by a certain person. In the early sessions this would immediately become a huge issue of conflict. I always comforted anyone who had been hit. (This was a very soft sponge ball and it was more a loss of dignity and security that was the issue, rather than any actual physical hurt.) This mothering response of mine quickly changed Vera's position. She realized that she was not hurt at all and that actually she was strong and still able to do lots of things. She got to the stage where even when the ball bounced on her head, she would laugh and say: 'We're not dead yet, we'll survive'. Holly benefited from her friend's new-found courage, which validated the worth of what we were doing together. Soon she was able to tell her son and be proud of her achievements in the group instead of denigrating it.

Of course the progression was not chronological because of the short-term memory loss, neither of them would remember anything about the group from week to week in the early sessions. Having left them very active and full of life and fun at the end of a session, I was horrified to return the next week to find two people, pale and unfocused with no memory of me at all, or of the activity we had enjoyed together. They would often be angry and disorientated, saying 'Something's going on here'. They did not know what it was but they described it as a deception of some kind. 'It might look all right on the surface,' they said but then they implied that it was a front for something much more sinister.

Trying to accept a realistic view of the illness and work with hope and positive appreciation of what they could achieve in the here and now, created a kind of balancing act in the group work and my relationship with them. In these early days I found that my movement mime, reminding them about how skilful they were with the ball, became the memory key. This was the concrete reminder even before they could remember and associate my face. My movement connected with the words, located the activity. Once they had this, then they were usually the first into the group. Gradually over the weeks my face also became the key so they would wave excitedly as they saw me through the window. They were then able to anticipate the activity and keep it in place while they went into the circle. This was a delight to me, as I would often find myself rushing around trying to assemble a group of people, most of whom would have no remembrance of the identity of such a group or any idea of place. Once Holly and Vera carried this knowledge and got irritated with the others who were often late, I was able to move more into the background. Although names were never remembered, the people and the group had become associated with the activity. From the little island of the twosome, a wider connection had been made with the rest of the community. If we sat together in the circle and began to play and talk about things that had happened in the week, this movement activity began to draw the others in. The memory networks seemed to be located in a connection between the movement activity and the holding, spatial form of the circle. When this was linked to the eye gaze and response of the people in the circle to those beyond, it seemed that the physical structure needed only two or three people, actively initiating contact, to attract others into the group. The friendship between the two, which had been unusual in this population, seemed to reach out to others. It reminded them of the possibility of rela-tionship. Momentary associations appeared and even glimpses of romance between group members. This was always picked up on and joked about. There was a noticeable increase in awareness of each other, shown by help offered and an alertness to the needs of other members of the group. This demonstrated the marked change in people who had initially not even been aware that someone else was even sitting beside them.

The ending of the session was always a test. It showed clearly that the group itself had created a safe, well-attached sense of place. This was con-trasted by the anxiety and fear of disintegration which came up when they suddenly realized they had to go somewhere else. What was 'there?' where they were staying, for example, was an unknown quantity. The idea that they lived in a room in the same building had no located meaning (Bowlby 1988). This always brought up anxiety for Vera, who would ask how was she going to get home to her mother. Holly would often laugh, saying she didn't have a clue where she was but it didn't matter because she always went to the police station when she got lost and she got a good cup of tea there. Vera would then agree that this was a good plan and if I could organize a cup of tea for everyone, this had a very stabilizing effect of locating time and place.

It was as if the circle had become a crucible that contained their identity and their stories. Here the fragments of memories of friends and family, games, joys and sorrows acquired a solid reality where they were again themselves.

A special farewell

A fact of working with this population will be that people die. Because of having individual time allotted, I found myself privileged to be able to work with a client when she was dying (Kubler Ross 1969). She had been a loyal and enthusiastic member of the group and when she was well had been on occasions able to dance with me in the circle. In the last weeks of her life when she was propped up in bed, I would spend regular sessions with her. We would hold the scarf and sway together and sing the songs. I would remind her of the dance and the group. At last when she was seemingly lying in a coma, I continued the work. I would put the scarf in her hands and began to talk to her and sing. On a special occasion on the day before she died, her bright blue eyes suddenly opened wide and she said: 'It's so very beautiful, this time for me, thank you so much for dancing with me...so beautiful...so very beautiful'. Her carer, who had been very distressed, also became involved. It seemed to give her a lot of comfort that her client was so peaceful and happy in connecting with such simple movements and song, when she herself had felt very helpless to do anything for her. She was able to continue singing with her when I was not there.

Conclusion

Working as a dance movement therapist with people with neural damage has shown me very clearly the fundamental nature of integration of mind and body. The third and synthesizing ingredient of the process of being human can be described variously as selfhood, emotional body, or spirit, with equal validity. We are essentially creatures who search for meaning. What actually takes place as 'healing' when all these aspects are enabled to integrate, accommodates science, humanism and spirituality. I feel that as a creative therapist I have been given the privileged position of being able to facilitate and witness this fusion on many occasions. The healing pattern in my clients and that in myself is interchangeable. In quantum terms we are a part of the whole in process (Bohm 1992). I feel a sense of optimism that I seem to be walking across a bridge, which spans scientific and therapeutic process. Somewhere in this transitional space is the synthesis necessary to span the discoveries from the journey between the Newtonian and Quantum worlds (Penrose 1995). In multidisciplinary co-operation, I believe we shall be able to find a positive way forward for a better quality of life for clients with dementia, clinicians and therapists.

Further information on Pilots, Projects and Reports can be obtained from the author at: 45 Savernake Road, London NW3 2JU. These include Pilot with older people in Camden, Pilot for The Rescue foundation, Movement and dance project for children with brain injury. Trauma work with The Dandelion Trust.

References

Achterberg, J., Dossey, B. and Kolkmeier, L. (1994) *Rituals of Healing*. New York: Bantam.

Ahmed, I. (1995) 'Pharmacological treatment of behavioural symptoms of Alzheimer's dementia: a review and a possible strategy.' *Clinical Gerontologist 16*, 1, 3–14.

Aigen, K. (1996) *Being in Music: Foundations of Nordoff–Robbins Music*. St Louis, MO: MMB Music.

Aldridge, A. (1995) 'Music therapy and the treatment of Alzheimer's disease.' *Clinical Gerontologist 16*, 1, 41–57.

Aldridge, D. (1995) 'Music therapy and the treatment of Alzheimer's disease.' Clinical Gerontologist *16*, 1, 41–57.

Aldridge, D. (1989) 'Music, communication and medicine: discussion paper.' *Journal of the Royal Society of Medicine 82*, 12, 743–746.

Aldridge, D. (1990) 'The development of a research strategy for music therapists in a hospital setting.' *The Arts in Psychotherapy 17*, 231–237.

Aldridge, D. (1991a) 'Aesthetics and the individual in the practice of medical research: a discussion paper.' *Journal of the Royal Society of Medicine 84*, 147–150.

Aldridge, D. (1991b) 'Creativity and consciousness: music therapy in intensive care.' *Arts in Psychotherapy 18*, 4, 359–362.

Aldridge, D. (1992) 'The needs of individual patients in clinical research.' *Advances 8*, 4, 58–65.

Aldridge, D. (1993a) 'Music and Alzheimer's disease – assessment and therapy: a discussion paper.' *Journal of the Royal Society of Medicine 86*, 93–95.

Aldridge, D. (1993b) 'The music of the body: music therapy in medical settings.' *Advances 9*, 1, 17–35.

Aldridge, D. (1993c) 'Artists or psychotherapists?' *The Arts in Psychotherapy 20*, 199–200.

Aldridge, D. (1994) 'Alzheimer's disease: rhythm, timing and music as therapy.' *Biomedical and Pharmocotherapy 48*, 7, 275–281.

Aldridge, D. (1996) *Music Therapy Research and Practice in Medicine: From Out of the Silence*. London: Jessica Kingsley Publishers.

Aldridge, D. (1998a) *Suicide: The Tragedy of Hopelessness*. London: Jessica Kingsley Publishers.

Aldridge, D. (1998b) 'Music therapy and the treatment of Alzheimer's disease.' *Journal of Clinical Geropsychology 4*, 1, 17–30.

Aldridge, D. (2000) *Spirituality, Healing and Medicine: Return to the Silence*. London: Jessica Kingsley Publishers.

Aldridge, D. and Aldridge, G. (1992) 'Two epistemologies: music therapy and medicine in the treatment of dementia.' *The Arts in Psychotherapy 19*, 243–255.

Aldridge, D. and Brandt, G. (1991) 'Music therapy and Alzheimer's disease.' *Journal of British Music Therapy 5*, 2, 28–63.

Aldridge, D., Brandt, G. and Wohler, D. (1989) 'Towards a common language among the creative art therapies.' *The Arts in Psychotherapy 17*, 189–195.

Aldridge, D., Gustorff, D. and Hannich, H. (1990) 'Where am I? Music therapy applied to coma patients [editorial].' *Journal of the Royal Society of Medicine 83*, 6, 345–346.

Allison, D. (1992) 'Profile of the Australian music therapist.' *Network*, 2–10.

Altenmüller, E. (1986) 'Brain correlates of cerebral music processing.' *European Archives of Psychiatry 235*, 342–354.

Alzheimer's Disease and Related Disorders Association (1998) *Alzheimer's Disease Fact Sheet*. Chicago: Alzheimer's Disease and Related Disorders Association, Inc.

American Music Therapy Association (AMTA) (1998) 'A descriptive statistical profile of 1998 AMTA membership.' (unpublished manuscript) http://www.musictherapy.org

American Psychiatric Association (1994) *Diagnostic and Statistical Manual of Mental Disorders* (4th edn). Washington, DC: Task Force on DSM-IV.

Ansdell, G. (1995) *Music for Life: Aspects of Creative Music Therapy with Adult Clients*. London: Jessica Kingsley Publishers.

Aronson, M., Post, D. and Guastadisegni, P. (1993) 'Dementia, agitation, and care in the nursing home.' *Journal of the American Geriatrics Society 41*, 5, 507–512.

Augsburger, D. (1996) *Helping People Forgive*. Louisville, KY: Westminister John Knox Press.

Bar-On, D. (1989) 'Children of perpetrators of the Holocaust: working through one's own moral self.' *Psychiatry 53*, 229–245.

Bartlett, J. and Snelus, P. (1980) 'Lifespan memory for popular songs.' *American Journal of Psychology 93*, 3, 551–560.

Bartlett, J., Halpern, A. and Dowling, W. (1995) 'Recognition of familiar and unfamiliar melodies in normal aging and Alzheimer's disease.' *Memory and Cognition 23*, 5, 531–546.

Bayles, K., Boone, D. and Tomoeda, C. (1989) 'Differentiating Alzheimer's patients from the normal elderly and stroke patients with aphasia.' *Journal of Speech and Hearing Disorders 54*, 74–87.

Bayles, K., Tomoeda, C. and Rein, J. (1996) 'Phrase repetition in Alzheimer's disease: effect of meaning and length.' *Brain and Language 54*, 2, 246–261.

Beatty, W., Brumback, R. and Vonsattel, J. (1997a) 'Autopsy-proven Alzheimer's disease in a patient with dementia who retained musical skill in life.' *Archives of Neurology 54*, 12, 1448.

Beatty, W., Testa, J., English, S. and Winn, P. (1997b) 'Influences of clustering and switching on the verbal fluency performance of patients with Alzheimer's disease.' *Aging Neuropsychology and Cognition 4*, 4, 273–279.

Beatty, W., Winn, P., Adams, R., Allen, E., Wilson, D., Price, J., Olson, K., Dean, K. and Littleford, D. (1994) 'Preserved cognitive skills in dementia of the Alzheimer type.' *Archives of Neurology 51*, 10, 1040–1046.

Beatty, W., Zavadil, K., Bailly, R., Rixen, G. and Zavadil, L., Farnham, N. and Fisher, L. (1988) 'Preserved musical skill in a severely demented patient.' *International Journal of Clinical Neuropsychology 10*, 4, 158–164.

Beck, C. (1998) 'Psychosocial and behavioural interventions for Alzheimer's disease patients and their families.' *American Journal of Geriatric Psychiatry 6*, 2, S41–S48.

Becker, J., Mintun, M., Aleva, K., Wiseman, M., Nichols, T. and Dekosky, S. (1996) 'Compensatory reallocation of brain resources supporting verbal episodic memory in Alzheimer's disease.' *Neurology 46*, 3, 692–700.

Behrens, G. and Green, S. (1993) 'The ability to identify emotional content of solo improvisations performed vocally and on three different instruments.' *Psychology of Music 21*, 20–33.

Bender, M. and Cheston, R. (1997) 'Inhabitants of a lost kingdom: a model of the subjective experiences of dementia.' *Ageing and Society 17*, 513–532.

Benke, T., Bosch, S. and Andree, B. (1998) 'A study of emotional processing in Parkinson's disease.' *Brain and Cognition 38*, 1, 36–52.

Berman, I. (1981) 'Musical functioning, speech lateralization and the amusias.' *South African Medical Journal 59*, 78–81.

Boden, C. (1998) *Who will I be When I Die?* East Melbourne: HarperCollins.

Bohm, D. (1992) *Wholeness and the Implicate Order.* London: Routledge.

Bonder, B. (1994) 'Psychotherapy for individuals with Alzheimer's disease.' *Alzheimer's Disease and Associated Disorders 8*, 3, 75–81.

Botwinick, J. (1978) *Aging and Behavior*, 2nd edn. New York: Springer.

Bowlby, J. (1988) *A Secure Base: Clinical Applications of Attachment Theory.* London: Routledge.

Braben, L. (1992) 'A song for Mrs. Smith.' *Nursing Times 88*, 41, 54.

Bright, R. (1972) *Music in Geriatric Care.* New York: Musicgraphics.

Bright, R. (1981) *Practical Planning in Music Therapy for the Aged.* New York: Musicgraphics.

Bright, R. (1986) 'The use of music therapy and activities with demented patients who are deemed "difficult to manage." Special: the elderly uncooperative patient.' *Clinical Gerontologist 6*, 2, 131–144.

Bright, R. (1988) *Music Therapy and the Dementias.* St Louis, MO: MMB Music.

Bright, R. (1991) *Music in Geriatric Care: A Second Look.* New South Wales, Australia: Music Therapy Enterprises.

Bright, R. (1997) *Wholeness in Later Life.* London: Jessica Kingsley Publishers.

Brookmeyer, R., Gray, S. and Kawas, C. (1998) 'Projections of Alzheimer's disease in the United States and the public health impact of delaying disease onset.' *American Journal of Public Health 88*, 9, 1337–1342.

Brotons, M. and Pickett-Cooper, P. (1994) 'Preferences of Alzheimer's disease patients for music activities: singing, instruments, dance/movement, games, and composition/improvisation.' *Journal of Music Therapy 31*, 220–233.

Brotons, M. and Pickett-Cooper, P. (1996) 'The effect of music therapy intervention on agitation behaviours of Alzheimer's disease patients.' *Journal of Music Therapy 33*, 1, 2–18.

Brotons, M., Koger, S. and Pickett-Cooper, P. (1997) 'Music and dementias: a review of literature.' *Journal of Music Therapy 34*, 204–245.

Brown University [Long-Term Care Quality Letter] (1995) 'Cognitive decline in Alzheimer's disease linked to agitation, education.'(adapted from *Journal of Gerontology: Medical Sciences* 50A:M49–M55, 1995).

Bruscia, K. (1995) 'The boundaries of music therapy research.' In B. Wheeler (ed) *Music Therapy Research: Quantitative and Qualitative Perspectives.* Phoenixville, PA: Barcelona Publishers.

Brust, J. (1980) 'Music and language: musical alexia and agraphia.' *Brain 103*, 2, 367–392.

Brustrom, J. and Ober, B. (1996) 'Source memory for actions in Alzheimer's disease.' *Aging Neuropsychology and Cognition 3*, 1, 56–66.

Bryant, W. (1991) 'Creative group work with confused elderly people: a development of sensory integration therapy.' *British Journal of Occupational Therapy 54*, 5, 187–192.

Cameron, J. (1997) *The Vein of Gold.* London: Pan.

Canadian Association for Music Therapy (CAMT) (1996) 'Survey results.' Internet. http://www.musictherapy.com/

Carruth, E. (1997) 'The effects of singing and the spaced retrieval technique on improving face-name recognition in nursing home residents with memory loss.' *Journal of Music Therapy 34*, 165–186.

Casby, J. and Holm, M. (1994) 'The effect of music on repetitive disruptive vocalizations of persons with dementia.' *American Journal of Occupational Therapy 48*, 10, 883–889.

Chenery, H. (1996) 'Semantic priming in Alzheimer's dementia.' *Aphasiology 10*, 1, 1–20.

Cheston, R. (1998) 'Psychotherapeutic work with people with dementia: a review of the literature.' *British Journal of Medical Psychology 71*, 211–231.

Christie, M. (1992) 'Music therapy applications in a skilled and intermediate care nursing home facility: a clinical study.' *Activities, Adaptation and Aging 16*, 4, 69–87.

Christie, M. (1995) 'The influence of a highly participatory peer on motivating group behaviours of lower functioning persons who have probable Alzheimer's type dementia: a feasibility study.' *Music Therapy Perspectives 13*, 2, 91–96.

Clair, A. (1990) 'The need for supervision to manage behaviour in the elderly care home resident and the implications for music therapy practice.' *Music Therapy Perspectives 8*, 72–75.

Clair, A. (1991) 'Music therapy for a severely regressed person with a probable diagnosis of Alzheimer's disease.' In K. Bruscia (ed) *Case Studies in Music Therapy.* Phoenixville, PA: Barcelona Press.

Clair, A. (1996a) *Therapeutic Uses of Music for Older Adults.* Baltimore, MD: Health Professions Press.

Clair, A. (1996b) 'The effect of singing on alert responses in persons with late stage dementia.' *Journal of Music Therapy 33*, 234–247.

Clair, A. (1999) 'Wellness activities for the active music making and wellness project.' Unpublished manuscript, University of Kansas, Lawrence.

Clair, A. and Bernstein, B. (1990a) 'A preliminary study of music therapy programming for severely regressed persons with Alzheimer's-type dementia.' *Journal of Applied Gerontology 9*, 3, 299–311.

Clair, A. and Bernstein, B. (1990b) 'A comparison of singing, vibrotactile and nonvibrotactile instrumental playing responses in severely regressed persons with dementia of the Alzheimer's type.' *Journal of Music Therapy 27*, 3, 119–125.

Clair, A. and Bernstein, B. (1993) 'The preference for vibrotactile versus auditory stimuli in severely regressed persons with dementia of the Alzheimer's type compared to those with dementia due to alcohol abuse.' *Music Therapy Perspectives 11*, 24–27.

Clair, A. and Bernstein, B. (1994) 'The effect of no music, stimulative background music and sedative background music on agitation behaviours in persons with severe dementia.' *Activities, Adaptation and Aging 19*, 1, 61–70.

Clair, A. and Ebberts, A. (1997) 'The effects of music therapy on interactions between family caregivers and their care receivers with late stage dementia.' *Journal of Music Therapy 34*, 148–164.

Clair, A., Bernstein, B. and Johnson, G. (1995) 'Rhythm playing characteristics in persons with severe dementia including those with probable Alzheimer's type.' *Journal of Music Therapy 32*, 2, 113–131.

Clair, A., Tebb, S. and Bernstein, B. (1993) 'The effects of socialization and music therapy intervention on self-esteem and loneliness in spouse caregivers of those diagnosed with dementia of the Alzheimer's type: a pilot study.' *American Journal of Alzheimer's Disease and Related Disorders and Research 1*, 24–32.

Clark, M.E., Lipe, A.W. and Bilbrey, M. (1998) 'Use of music to decrease aggressive behaviours in people with dementia.' *Journal of Gerontological Nursing 24*, 7, 10–17.

Clayton, J. (1991) 'Let there be life: an approach to worship with Alzheimer's patients and their families.' *Journal of Pastoral Care 45*, 2, 177–179.

Clendaniel, B. P. and Fleishell, A. (1989) 'An Alzheimer day-care center for nursing home patients.' *American Journal of Nursing 89*, 944–945.

Cohen, D., Eisdorfer, C., Groelick, P., Paveza, G., Luchins, D., Freels, S., Ashforde, J., Semal, T., Levy, P. and Hirschman, R. (1993) 'Psychopathology associated with Alzheimer's disease and related disorders.' *Journal of Gerontology 48*, 6, 255–260.

Cohen, N. (1992) 'The effect of singing instruction on the speech production of neurologically impaired persons.' *Journal of Music Therapy 29*, 87–102.

Cohen, N. (1994) 'Speech and song: implications for music therapy.' *Music Therapy Perspectives 12*, 8–14.

Cohen, N. (1995a) 'The effect of musical cues on the nonpurposive speech of persons with aphasia.' *Journal of Music Therapy 32*, 46–57.

Cohen, N. (1995b) 'The effect of vocal instruction and Visi-Pitch™ feedback on the speech of persons with neurogenic communication disorders: two case studies.' *Music Therapy Perspectives 13*, 70–75.

Cohen, N. and Masse, R. (1993) 'The application of singing and rhythmic instruction as a therapeutic intervention for persons with neurogenic communication disorders.' *Journal of Music Therapy 30*, 81–99.

Cohen, N. and Squire, L. (1980) 'Preserved learning and retention of pattern-analyzing skill in amnesia: dissociation of knowing how and knowing that.' *Science 210*, 207–210.

Cohen-Mansfield, J. (1992) 'Observational data on time use and behaviour problems in the nursing home.' *Journal of Applied Gerontology 11*, 1, 111–121.

Cohen-Mansfield, J. (1996) 'Behavioural and mood evaluations: assessment of agitation.' *International Psychogeriatrics 8*, 2, 233–245.

Cohen-Mansfield, J. and Billig, N. (1986) 'Agitated behaviours in the elderly: a conceptual review.' *Journal of the American Geriatrics Society 34*, 711–721.

Cohen-Mansfield, J. and Marx, M. (1990) 'The relationship between sleep disturbances and agitation in a nursing home.' *Journal of Aging and Health 2*, 1, 42–57.

Cohen-Mansfield, J., Marx, M. and Rosenthal, A. (1989) 'A description of agitation in a nursing home.' *Journal of Gerontology: Medical Science 44*, M77–M84.

Cohen-Mansfield, J., Marx, M. and Rosenthal, A. (1990) 'Dementia and agitation: how are they related?' *Psychology and Aging 5*, 1, 3–8.

Collette, F., VanderLinden, M., Bechet, S., Belleville, S. and Salmon, E. (1998) 'Working memory deficits in Alzheimer's disease.' *Brain and Cognition 37*, 1, 147–149.

Cooper, J. (1991) 'Songs that soothe.' *New Zealand Nursing Journal 84*, 3, 22–23.

Crisp, J. (1995) 'Making sense of the stories that people with Alzheimer's tell: a journey with my mother.' *Nursing Inquiry 2*, 133–140.

Crystal, H., Grober, E. and Masur, D. (1989) 'Preservation of musical memory in Alzheimer's disease.' *Journal of Neurology, Neurosurgery, and Psychiatry 52*, 1415–1416.

Csordas, T. (1983) 'The rhetoric of transformation in ritual healing.' *Culture, Medicine and Psychiatry 7*, 4, 333–75.

Dalai Lama (1996) '"Message" to "Sterben, Tod und Leben" ["Dying, Death and Living"].' International and Interdisciplinary Kongress, Munich, Germany, 21–24 November, Kongress Programme, p.5.

Dalessio, D. (1984) 'Maurice Ravel and Alzheimer's disease.' *Journal of the American Medical Association 252*, 24, 3412–3413.

Damasio, A. (1994) *Descartes' Error: Emotion, Reason and the Human Brain.* New York: Grosset/Putnam Books. London: Picador.

Damasio, A. (2000) *The Feeling of What Happens.* London: Heinemann.

Daniel, J. (1996) *Looking After: A Son's Memoir.* Washington, DC: Counterpoint.

Darrow, A., Johnson, C. and Ollenberger, T. (1994) 'The effect of participation in an intergenerational choir on teens' and older persons' cross-age attitudes.' *Journal of Music Therapy 31*, 119–134.

Davis, L., Buckwalter, K. and Burgio, L. (1997) 'Measuring problem behaviours in dementia: developing a methodological approach.' *Advances in Nursing Science 20*, 1, 40–56.

Davis, R. (1989) *My Journey into Alzheimer's Disease.* Amersham: Scripture Press.

Denney, A. (1997) 'Quiet music: an intervention for mealtime agitation?' *Journal of Gerontological Nursing 23*, 7, 16–23.

Dick, M., Nielson, K., Beth, R., Shankle, W. and Cotman, C. (1995) 'Acquisition and long-term retention of a fine motor skill in Alzheimer's disease.' *Brain and Cognition 29*, 3, 294–306.

Dienstfrey, H. (1999) 'Disclosure and health: an interview with James W. Pennebaker.' *Advances 15*, 161–195.

Dossey, L. (1993) *Healing Words: The Power of Prayer and the Practice of Medicine.* San Francisco, CA: Harper.

Dowling, W. and Harwood, J. (1986) *Music and Cognition.* New York: Academic Press.

Drieschner, K. and Pioch, A. (1998) 'How music therapists adapt their methods to categories of clients and therapy settings: an empirical study.' Unpublished manuscript.

Droës, R. (1998) 'Kwaliteit van zorg en kwaliteit van leven bij dementie.' *Lecture Nationaal Congres Ouder Worden*, March.

Ellis, D. (1996) 'Coherence patterns in Alzheimer's discourse.' *Communication Research 23*, 4, 472–495.

Engelmann, I. (1995) 'Musiktherapie in psychiatrische Kliniken.' *Nervenarzt 66*, 217–224.

Erfer, T. (1993) 'Treating children with autism in the public school system.' In F. Levy (ed) *Dance and Other Expressive Art Therapies*. London: Routledge.

Fitzgerald-Cloutier, M. (1993) 'The use of music therapy to decrease wandering: an alternative to restraints.' *Music Therapy Perspectives 11*, 1, 32–36.

Folstein, M., Folstein, S. and McHugh, P. (1975) '"Mini-Mental State:" a practical method for grading the cognitive state of patients for the clinician.' *Journal of Psychiatric Research 12*, 189–198.

Forsell, Y., Jorm, A. and Winblad, B. (1998) 'The outcome of depression and dysthymia in a very elderly population: results from a three-year follow-up study.' *Aging and Mental Health 2*, 2, 100–104.

Foster, N. (1998) 'An examination of the facilitatory effect of music on recall, with special reference to dementia sufferers.' Unpublished PhD thesis, Royal Holloway College, University of London.

Fox, J. (1997) *Poetic Medicine*. New York: Jeremy P. Tarcher/Putnam.

Gabrielson, A. and Juslin, P. (1996) 'Emotional expression in music performance: between the performer's intention and the listener's experience.' *Psychology of Music 24*, 68–91.

Gaebler, H. and Hemsley, D. (1991) 'The assessment and short-term manipulation of affect in the severely demented.' *Behavioural Psychotherapy 19*, 145–156.

Gates, A. and Bradshaw, J. (1977) 'The role of cerebral hemispheres in music.' *Brain and Language 4*, 403–431.

Gates, G., Cobb, J., Linn, R., Rees, T., Wolf, P. and Dagostino, R. (1996) 'Central auditory dysfunction, cognitive dysfunction, and dementia in older people.' *Archives of Otolaryngology: Head and Neck Surgery 122*, 2, 161–167.

Gauthier, D. (1992) 'Vocal education: as short "chorus".' *Music Therapy Perspectives 10*, 105–109.

Gerdner, L. and Swanson, E. (1993) 'Effects of individualized music on confused and agitated elderly patients.' *Archives of Psychiatric Nursing 7*, 5, 284–291.

Gergen, K. (1997) 'Psycho-versus bio-medical therapy.' *Society 35*, 1, 24–27.

Geula, M. (1986) 'Activities for AD: music encourages self-expression.' *Alzheimer's Disease and Related Disorders Newsletter 6*, 2, 7.

Gibbons, A. (1977) 'Popular music preferences of elderly people.' *Journal of Music Therapy 14*, 4, 180–189.

Gibbons, A. and Heller, G. (1985) 'Music therapy in Handel's England.' *College Music Symposium 25*, 59–72.

Gilbert, J. (1977) 'Music therapy perspectives on death and dying.' *Journal of Music Therapy 14*, 4, 165–171.

Gilhooly, M. and Birren, J. (1986) 'Introduction.' In M.L.M. Gilhooly, S.H. Zarit and J.E. Birren (eds) *The Dementias: Policy and Management.* Englewood Cliffs, NJ: Prentice-Hall.

Glassman, L. (1983) 'The talent show: meeting the needs of the healthy elderly.' *Music Therapy 3*, 1, 82–93.

Glosser, G., Wiley, M. and Barnoski, E. (1998) 'Gestural communication in Alzheimer's disease.' *Journal of Clinical and Experimental Neuropsychology 20*, 1, 1–13.

Glynn, N. (1992) 'The music therapy assessment tool in Alzheimer's disease.' *Journal of Gerontological Nursing 18*, 1, 3–9.

Goddaer, J. and Abraham, I. (1994) 'Effects of relaxing music on agitation during meals among nursing home residents with severe cognitive impairment.' *Archives of Psychiatric Nursing 8*, 3, 150–158.

Goldberg, N. (1998) 'Interview with Dr. Larry Dossey.' *International Journal of Arts Medicine 5*, 2, 40–42.

Goldhagen, D. (1996) *Hitler's Willing Executioners: Ordinary Germans and the Holocaust.* New York: Alfred A. Knopf.

Goldsmith, M. (1996) *Hearing the Voice of People with Dementia: Opportunities and Obstacles.* London: Jessica Kingsley Publishers.

Griffiths, J. (1995) *Griefwork with the Person with Dementia: Is it Different in Nature?* Adelaide: NALAG Conference Proceedings.

Groene, R. (1993) 'Effectiveness of music therapy intervention with individuals having senile dementia of the Alzheimer's type.' *Journal of Music Therapy 30*, 3, 138–157.

Groene, R., Zapchenk, S., Marble, G. and Kantar, S. (1998) 'The effect of therapist and activity characteristics on the purposeful responses of probable Alzheimer's disease participants.' *Journal of Music Therapy 35*, 119–136.

Gunther, W., Giunta, R., Klages, U., Haag, C., Steinberg, R., Satzger, W., Jonitz, L. and Engel, R. (1993) 'Findings of electroencephalographic brain mapping in mild to moderate dementia of the Alzheimer type during resting, motor, and music perception conditions.' *Psychiatry Research, Neuroimaging 50*, 3, 163–176.

Gutt, C. (1996) 'Health and wellness in the community.' In J.M. Cookfair (ed) *Nursing Care in the Community.* St Louis, MO: Mosby.

Gwyther, L. and Strulowitz, S. (1998) 'Care-giver stress.' *Current Opinion in Psychiatry 11*, 4, 431–434.

Hall, G. and Buckwalter, K. (1987) 'Progressively lowered stress threshold: a conceptual model for care of adults with Alzheimer's disease.' *Archives of Psychiatric Nursing 1*, 399–406.

Hamilton-Smith, E. (1996) 'Enhanced lifestyle through optimal stimulus – or can dementia be successful ageing?' Keynote address to 1996 National Conference, Australian Association of Gerontology, Hobart, Australia.

Haneishi, E. (1999) 'The effects of music therapy voice treatment on speech and voice problems and mood of individuals with Parkinson's disease.' Unpublished Master's thesis, University of Kansas, Lawrence.

Hannaford, C. (1995) *Smart Moves. Why Learning is Not All in your Head.* Arlington, VA: Great Ocean.

Hanser, S. (1990) 'A music therapy strategy for depressed older adults in the community.' *Journal of Applied Gerontology 9*, 283–298.

Hanser, S. and Clair, A. (1995) 'Retrieving the losses of Alzheimer's disease for patients and caregivers with the aid of music.' In T. Wigram, B. Saperston and R. West (eds) *The Art and Science of Music Therapy: A Handbook.* Switzerland: Harwood Academic Publishers.

Hanson, N., Gfeller, K., Woodworth, G., Swanson, E. and Garand, L. (1996) 'A comparison of the effectiveness of differing types and difficulty of music activities in programming for older adults with Alzheimer's Disease and related disorders.' *Journal of Music Therapy 33*, 2, 93–123.

Harlan, J. (1993) 'The therapeutic value of art for persons with Alzheimer's disease and related disorders.' *Loss, Grief and Care 6*, 4, 99–106.

Harris, P. (1998) 'Listening to caregiving sons: misunderstood realities.' *Gerontologist 38*, 3, 342–352.

Heal, H. and Husband, H. (1998) 'Disclosing a diagnosis of dementia: is age a factor?' *Aging and Mental Health 2*, 2, 144–150.

Hendrie, H. (1998) 'Epidemiology of dementia and Alzheimer's disease.' *American Journal of Geriatric Psychiatry 6*, 2, S3–S18.

Henson, R. (1988) 'Maurice Ravel's illness: a tragedy of lost creativity.' *British Medical Journal of Clinical Research 296*, 6636, 1585–1588.

Hesse, H. (1973) *The Glass Bead Game.* Harmondsworth: Penguin.

Holden, U. (1987) *Neuropsychology and Ageing.* London: Croom Helm.

Holliday, L. (1995) *Children in the Holocaust and World War II: Their Secret Diaries.* New York: Pocket Books.

Hopkins, R., Rindlisbacher, P. and Grant, N. (1992) 'An investigation of the sundowning syndrome and ambient light.' *American Journal of Alzheimer's Care and Related Disorders and Research 3*, 22–27.

Jacome, D. (1984) 'Aphasia with elation, hypermusia, musicophilia and compulsive whistling.' *Journal of Neurology Neurosurgery and Psychiatry 47*, 3, 308–310.

Johnson, C., Lahey, P. and Shore, A. (1992) 'An exploration of creative arts therapeutic group work on an Alzheimer's unit.' *The Arts in Psychotherapy 19*, 269–277.

Jonas, J. (1991) 'Preferences of elderly music listeners residing in nursing homes for art music, traditional jazz, popular music of today, and country music.' *Journal of Music Therapy 28*, 3, 149–160.

Jungels, D. and Belcher, J. (1985) '"My cheeks are rosy anyway: I can't be dead." A multi-arts programme at a mental institution.' In N. Weisberg and R. Wilder (eds) *Creative Arts with Older Adults: A Sourcebook.* New York: Human Sciences Press.

Kamar, O. (1997) 'Light and death: art therapy with a patient with Alzheimer's disease.' *American Journal of Art Therapy 35*, 4, 118–124.

Kane, R.L., Klein, S.J., Bernstein, L., Rothenberg, R. and Wales, J. (1985) 'Hospice role in alleviating the emotional stress of terminal patients and their families.' *Medical Care 23*, 3, 189–197.

Kartman, L. (1990) 'Fun and entertainment: one aspect of making meaningful music for the elderly.' *Activities, Adaptation and Aging 14*, 4, 39–44.

Keady, J. and Nolan, M. (1995) 'A stitch in time: facilitating proactive interventions with dementia care givers.' *Journal of Psychiatric and Mental Health Nursing 2*, 33–40.

Kellar, L. and Bever, T. (1980) 'Hemispheric asymmetries in the perception of musical intervals as a function of musical experience.' *Brain and Language 10*, 24–38.

Khachaturian, Z. and Radebaugh, T. (1996) *Alzheimer's Disease: Causes, Diagnosis, Treatment, and Care.* Boca Raton, FL: CRC Press.

Kidd, G., Boltz, M. and Jones, M. (1984) 'Some effects of rhythmic context on melody recognition.' *American Journal of Psychology 97*, 2, 153–173.

Kierkegaard, S. (1988 [1845]) *Stages on Life's Way.* Edited and translated by Howard V. Hong and Edna H. Hong. Princeton, NJ: Princeton University Press.

Killick, J. (1994) *Please Give Me Back My Personality!* Stirling: Dementia Services Development Centre, University of Stirling.

Killick, J. (1996) 'Attitudes to the end.' Paper presented to sixth Alzheimer Europe Annual Meeting, Warsaw.

Killick, J. (1998) 'A matter of the life and death of the mind: creative writing with dementia sufferers.' In C. Hunt and F. Sampson (eds) *The Self on the Page.* London: Jessica Kingsley Publishers.

Killick, J. (1999) 'Pathways through pain: a cautionary tale.' *Journal of Dementia Care 7*, 1, 22–24.

Kitwood, T. (1997) *Dementia Reconsidered: The Person Comes First.* Buckingham: Open University Press.

Kitwood, T. and Bredin, K. (1992) 'Towards a theory of dementia care: personhood and well-being.' *Ageing and Society 13*, 269–287.

Kneafsey, R. (1997) 'The therapeutic use of music in a care of the elderly setting: a literature review.' *Journal of Clinical Nursing 6*, 341–346.

Knill, P. (1995) 'The place of beauty in therapy and the arts.' *The Arts in Psychotherapy 22*, 1–7.

Knott, R., Patterson, K. and Hodges, J. (1997) 'Lexical and semantic binding effects in short-term memory: evidence from semantic dementia.' *Cognitive Neuropsychology 14*, 8, 1165–1218.

Koh, I. (1998) 'The effect of singing on the facial expression of elderly individuals in hospice/palliative care: three case studies.' Unpublished Master's thesis, University of Kansas, Lawrence.

Korb, C. (1997) 'The influence of music therapy on patients with a diagnosed dementia.' *Canadian Journal of Music Therapy 5*, 1, 26–54.

Kubler Ross, E. (1969) *On Death and Dying.* London: Macmillan.

Langer, S. (1953) *Feeling and Form.* New York: Scribner's.

Larner, G. (1998) 'Through a glass darkly.' *Theory and Psychology 8*, 4, 549–572.

Larson, E. (1998) 'Management of Alzheimer's disease in a primary care setting.' *American Journal of Geriatric Psychiatry 6*, 2, S34–S40.

Leventhal, M. (1979) 'Structure in dance therapy: a model for personality integration.' *CORD Dance Research Annual 10*, 173–182.

Leventhal, M. (1980) *Movement and Growth: Dance Therapy for the Special Child.* New York: New York University Press.

Levitt, S. (1995) *Treatment of Cerebral Palsy and Motor Delay.* London: Blackwell Science.

Lindenmuth, G., Patel, M. and Chang, P. (1992) 'Effects of music on sleep in healthy elderly and subjects with senile dementia of the Alzheimer's type.' *American Journal of Alzheimer's Care and Related Disorders and Research 2*, 13–20.

Linn, D. and Linn, M. (1978) *Healing Life's Hurts*. New York: Paulist Press.

Lipe, A. (1991) 'Using music therapy to enhance the quality of life in a client with Alzheimer's dementia: a case study.' *Music Therapy Perspectives 9*, 102–105.

Lipe, A. (1992) 'Music debate.' *Journal of Gerontological Nursing 18*, 7, 3–4.

Lipe, A. (1995) 'The use of music performance tasks in the assessment of cognitive functioning among older adults with dementia.' *Journal of Music Therapy 32*, 3, 137–151.

Lloyd, S. (1992) 'Finding the key: nursing narratives.' *Nursing Times 88*, 32, 48.

Lochner, C. and Stevenson, R. (1988) 'Music as a bridge to wholeness.' *Death Studies 12*, 175–180.

Longino, C., Soldo, B. and Manton, K. (1990) 'Demography of aging in the United States.' In K.F. Ferraro (ed) *Gerontology: Perspectives and Issues*. New York: Springer.

Lord, T. and Garner, J. (1993) 'Effects of music on Alzheimer's patients.' *Perceptual and Motor Skills 76*, 451–455.

Lucero, M., Hutchinson, S., Leger-Krall, S. and Wilson, H. (1993) 'Wandering in Alzheimer's dementia patients.' *Clinical Nursing Research 2*, 2, 160–175.

McCloskey, L. (1985) 'Music and the frail elderly.' *Activities, Adaptation and Aging 7*, 2, 73–75.

McCloskey, L. (1990) 'The silent heart sings. Special Issue: counseling and therapy for elders.' *Generations 14*, 1, 63–65.

McGowin, D.F. (1993) *Living in the Labyrinth*. Cambridge: Mainsail Press.

McGowin, D.F. (1994) *Living in the Labyrinth: A Personal Journey through the Maze of Alzheimer's*. New York: Dell.

McLean, B. (1993) 'Music debates continues.' *Journal of Gerontological Nursing 19*, 2, 5–6.

Mahler, M., Pine, F. and Bergman, A. (1975) *The Psychological Birth of the Human Infant*. New York: Basic Books.

Mandel, S. (1991) 'Music therapy in the hospice: "Musicalive".' *Palliative Medicine 5*, 155–160.

Mango, C. (1992) 'Emma: art therapy illustrating personal and universal images of loss.' *Omega Journal of Death and Dying 25*, 4, 259–269.

Martinson, I. (1992) 'Response to "chronic sorrow": a lifespan concept.' *Scholarly Inquiry for Nursing Practice: An International Journal 6*, 1, 41–48.

Merritt, S. (1998) 'Breaking the silence: GIM and the Nazi legacy.' Unpublished doctoral dissertation, Summit University of Louisiana.

Meyer, L. (1956) *Emotion and Meaning in Music*. Chicago: University of Chicago Press.

Miesen, B. and Jones, G. (1997) 'Psychic pain resurfacing in dementia: from new to past trauma?' In L. Hunt, M. Marshall and C. Rowlings (eds) *Past Trauma in Late Life: European Perspectives on Therapeutic Work with Older People*. London: Jessica Kingsley Publishers.

Miller, P. (1994) *Writing your Life*. St Leonards, Australia: Allen and Unwin.

Miller, R. (1998) 'Epistemology and psychotherapy data: the unspeakable, unbearable, horrible truth.' *Clinical Psychology: Science and Practice 5*, 2, 242–250.

Mills, M. (1997) 'Narrative identity and dementia: a study of emotion and narrative in older people with dementia.' *Ageing and Society 17*, 673–698.

Mohacsy, I. (1995) 'Nonverbal communication and its place in the therapy session.' *The Arts in Psychotherapy 221*, 31–38.

Moore, R., Staum, M. and Brotons, M. (1992) 'Music preferences of the elderly: repertoire, vocal ranges, tempos and accompaniments for singing.' *Journal of Music Therapy 29*, 236–252.

Morgan, O. and Tilluckdharry, R. (1982) 'Presentation of singing function in severe aphasia.' *West Indian Medical Journal 31*, 159–161.

Morris, M. (1986) 'Music and movement for the elderly.' *NursingTimes 82*, 8, 44–45.

Munro, S. (1994) *Music Therapy in Palliative/Hospice Care.* St Louis, MO: MMB Music.

Neijmeijer, L., Wijgert, J. van der and Hutschemaekers, G. (1996) *Beroep: vaktherapeut/ vakbegeleider: een verkennend onderzoek naar persoon, werk en werkplek van vaktherapeuten en vakbegeleiders in de gezondheidszorg.* Utrecht: Nederlands Centrum Geestelijke Volksgezondheid.

Newman, S. and Ward, C. (1993) 'An observational study of intergenerational activities and behaviour change in dementing elders at adult day care centers.' *International Journal of Aging and Human Development 36*, 4, 321–333.

Nieuwenhuizen, N. and Broersen, M. (1998) 'Muziek therapie: waar woorden te koet schieien.' *Leidraad Psychogeratie,* B4, 100–103.

Norberg, A., Melin, E. and Asplund, K. (1986) 'Reactions to music, touch and object presentation in the final stage of dementia: an exploratory study.' *International Journal of Nursing Studies 23*, 4, 315–323.

Nordoff, P. and Robbins, C. (1971) *Therapy in Music for Handicapped Children.* London: Gollancz.

Nordoff, P. and Robbins, C. (1977) *Creative Music Therapy.* New York: John Day.

Olderog-Millard, K.A. and Smith, J.M. (1989) 'The influence of group singing on the behaviour of Alzheimer's disease patients.' *Journal of Music Therapy 26*, 58–70.

Orange, J., Van Gennep, K., Miller, L. and Johnson, A. (1998) 'Resolution of communication breakdown in dementia of the Alzheimer's type: a longitudinal study.' *Journal of Applied Communication Research 26*, 1, 120–138.

Ortiz, J. (1997) *The Tao of Music.* York Beach, ME: Samuel Weiser.

Owings, A. (1995) *Frauen: German Women Recall the Third Reich.* New Brunswick, NJ: Rutgers University.

Palmer, M. (1977) 'Music therapy in a comprehensive programme of treatment and rehabilitation for the geriatric resident.' *Journal of Music Therapy 14*, 4, 190–197.

Palmer, M. (1983) 'Music therapy in a comprehensive programme of treatment and rehabilitation for the geriatric resident.' *Activities, Adaptation and Aging 3*, 3, 53–59.

Palmer, M. (1989) 'Music therapy in gerontology: a review and a projection. National Association for Music Therapy California Symposium on Clinical Practices.' (1987, Costa Mesa, CA). *Music Therapy Perspectives 6*, 52–56.

Penrose, R. (1995) *Shadows of the Mind.* London: Vintage.

Polk, M. and Kerstesz, A. (1993) 'Music and language in degenerative disease of the brain.' *Brain and Cognition 22*, 1, 98–117.

Pollack, N. and Namazi, K. (1992) 'The effect of music participation on the social behaviour of Alzheimer's disease patients.' *Journal of Music Therapy 29*, 1, 54–67.

Pomeroy, V. (1993) 'The effect of physiotherapy input on mobility skills of elderly people with severe dementing illness.' *Clinical Rehabilitation 7*, 163–170.

Pomeroy, V. (1994) 'Immobility and severe dementia: when is physiotherapy appropriate?' *Clinical Rehabilitation 8*, 226–232.

Post, S. (1995) *The Moral Challenge of Alzheimer's Disease.* Baltimore, MD: Johns Hopkins University Press.

Pot, A., Deeg, D. and Van Dyck, R. (1997) 'Psychological well-being of informal caregivers of elderly people with dementia: changes over time.' *Aging and Mental Health 1*, 3, 261–268.

Povel, D. (1984) 'A theoretical framework for rhythm perception.' *Psychological Research 45*, 315–337.

Prange, P. (1990) 'Categories of music therapy at Judson Retirement Community.' *Music Therapy Perspectives 8*, 88–89.

Prickett, C. (1988) 'Music therapy for the aged.' In C. Furman (ed) *Effectiveness of Music Therapy Procedures: Documentation of Research and Clinical Practice.* Silver Spring, MD: National Association for Music Therapy.

Prickett, C. (1996) 'Music therapy as a part of older people's lives.' In C. Furman (ed) *Effectiveness of Music Therapy Procedures: Documentation of Research and Clinical Practice,* 2nd edn. Washington, DC: National Association for Music Therapy.

Prickett, C. and Moore, R. (1991) 'The use of music to aid memory of Alzheimer's patients.' *Journal of Music Therapy 28*, 2, 101–110.

Prinsley, D. (1986) 'Music therapy in geriatric care.' *Australian Nurses Journal 15*, 9, 48–49.

Radocy, R. and Boyle, J. (1979) *Psychological Foundations of Musical Behavior.* Springfield, IL: Charles C. Thomas.

Ragneskog, H., Brane, G., Karlsson, I. and Kihlgren, M. (1996a) 'Influence of dinner music on food intake and symptoms common in dementia.' *Scandinavian Journal of Caring Science 10*, 11–17.

Ragneskog, H., Kihlgren, M., Karlsson, I. and Norberg, A. (1996b) 'Dinner music for demented patients: analysis of video-recorded observations.' *Clinical Nursing Research 5*, 3, 262–282.

Ramig, L.O., Bonitati, C.M., Lemke, J.H. and Horri, Y. (1994) 'Voice treatment for patients with Parkinson disease: development of an approach and preliminary efficacy data.' *Journal of Medical Speech-Language Pathology 2*, 191–209.

Raskind, M. (1998) 'The clinical interface of depression and dementia.' *Journal of Clinical Psychiatry 59*, 9–12.

Reisberg, B, Fernis, S. H., De Leon, M. J. and Crook, T. (1982) 'The global deterioration scale for assessment of primary degenerative dementia.' *American Journal of Psychiatry 139*, 9, 1136–1139.

Richards, M. (1986) *Let's Do it Again.* San Francisco, CA: Richard's Institute.

Richarz, B. (1997) 'Considerations to the psychosomatics of Alzheimer's disease.' *Dynamische Psychiatrie 30*, 5–6, 340–355.

Rickert, E., Duke, L., Putzke, J., Marson, D. and Graham, K. (1998) 'Early stage Alzheimer's disease disrupts encoding of contextual information.' *Aging Neuropsychology and Cognition 5*, 1, 73–81.

Roberts, U. (1994) *Starke Mutter, Ferne Väter. [Strong Mothers, Absent Fathers].* Frankfurt am Main: Fischer Taschenbuch Verlag.

Roose-Evans, J. (1994) *Passages of the Soul: Rediscovering the Importance of Rituals in Everyday Life.* Shaftesbury: Element.

Rose, S. (1992) *The Making of Memory.* New York: Anchor.

Rosling, L.K. and Kitchen, J. (1992) 'Music and drawing with institutionalized elderly. Miniconference in Music and Geriatrics (1990, Coquitlam, Canada).' *Activities, Adaptation and Aging 17*, 2, 27–38.

Rudy, J. and Sutherland, R. (1994) 'The memory-coherence problem, configural associations, and the hippocampal system.' In D.L. Schacter and E. Tulving (eds) *Memory Systems.* Cambridge, MA: MIT Press.

Rusted, J., Marsh, R., Bledski, L. and Sheppard, L. (1997) 'Alzheimer patients' use of auditory and olfactory cues to aid verbal memory.' *Aging and Mental Health 1*, 4, 364–371.

Sacks, O.W. (1999) 'Music and the brain.' In C.M. Tomaino (ed) *Clinical Applications of Music in Neurologic Rehabilitation.* St Louis, MO: MMB Press.

Sacks, O. and Tomaino, C. (1991) 'Music and neurological disorder.' *International Journal of Arts Medicine 1*, 1, 10–12.

Sambandham, M. and Schirm, V. (1995) 'Music as a nursing intervention for residents with Alzheimer's disease in long-term care.' *Geriatric Nursing 16*, 2, 79–82.

Sandel, S. and Johnson, D. (1983) 'Structure and process of the nascent group: dance therapy with chronic patients.' *Arts in Psychotherapy 10*, 131–140.

Sandel, S. and Johnson, D. (1987) *Waiting at the Gate: Creativity and Hope in the Nursing Home.* New York: Harworth.

Saunders, C. (1965) 'Watch with me.' Reprinted from *Nursing Times,* 26 November.

Schachtel, E. (1946) 'On memory and childhood amnesia.' *Psychiatry 10*, 1–26.

Schacter, D.L. (1996) *Searching for Memory.* New York: Basic Books.

Schafer, W. (1992) *Stress Management for Wellness,* 2nd edn. Fort Worth, TX: Harcourt Brace.

Schroeder-Sheker, T. (1993) 'Music for the dying: a personal account of the new field of music thanatology – history, theories, and clinical narratives.' *Advances 9*, 36–48.

Schullian, D. and Schoen, M. (1948) *Music and Medicine.* New York: Henry Schuman.

Scruggs, S. (1991) 'The effects of structured music activities versus contingent music listening with verbal prompt on wandering behavior and cognition in geriatric patients with Alzheimer's disease.' Unpublished Master's thesis, Florida State University, Tallahassee.

Sears, W. (1966) 'Processes in music therapy.' In E.T. Gaston (ed) *Music in Therapy.* Lawrence, KS: Allen Press.

Segal, R. (1990) 'Helping older mentally retarded persons expand their socialization skills through the use of expressive therapies. Special issue: activities with developmentally disabled elderly and older adults.' *Activities, Adaptation and Aging 15*, 1–2, 99–109.

Semon, R. (1921) *The Mneme*. London: Allen and Unwin.

Shively, C. and Henkin, L. (1986) 'Music and movement therapy with Alzheimer's victims.' *Music Therapy Perspectives 3*, 56–58.

Silber, F. and Hes, J. (1995) 'The use of songwriting with patients diagnosed with Alzheimer's disease.' *Music Therapy Perspectives 13*, 1, 31–34.

Sloboda, J. (1989) 'Music as a language.' In F.R. Wilson and F.L. Roehmann (eds) *Music and Child Development*. St Louis, MO: MMB Music.

Smeijsters, H. (1993) 'Music therapy in the Netherlands.' In C.D. Maranto (ed) *Music Therapy: International Perspectives*. Pipersville, PA: Jeffrey Books.

Smeijsters, H. (1995) *Handboek Muziektherapie*. Melos: Heerlen.

Smeijsters, H. (1997) 'Musiktherapie bei Alzheimerpatienten. Eine Meta-Analyse von Forschungsergebnissen. [Music therapy in the treatment of Alzheimer Patient. A meta-analysis of research results].' *Musiktherapeutische Umschau 1997*, 4, 268–283.

Smith, B. (1992) 'Treatment of dementia: healing through cultural arts.' *Pride Institute Journal of Long Term Home Health Care 11*, 3, 37–45.

Smith, D. (1990) 'Therapeutic treatment effectiveness as documented in the gerontology literature: implications for music therapy.' *Music Therapy Perspectives 8*, 36–40.

Smith, D. (1999) 'The civilizing process and the history of sexuality: comparing Norbert Elias and Michael Foucault.' *Theory and Society 28*, 79–100.

Smith, G. (1986) 'A comparison of the effects of three treatment interventions on cognitive functioning of Alzheimer patients.' *Music Therapy 6a*, 1, 41–56.

Smith, S. (1990) 'The unique power of music therapy benefits Alzheimer's patients.' *Activities, Adaptation and Aging 14*, 4, 59–63.

Smith-Marchese, K. (1994) 'The effects of participatory music on the reality orientation and sociability of Alzheimer's residents in a long-term care setting.' *Activities, Adaptation and Aging 18*, 2, 41–55.

Sparks, R.W. and Holland, A.L. (1976) 'Method: melodic infromation therapy for aphasia.' *Journal od Speech and Hearing Disorders 41*, 298–300.

Special Committee on Aging, United States Senate (1991) *Forever Young: Music and aging. Hearing before the Special Committee on Aging. United States Senate* (Serial no. 102–9). Washington, DC: US Government Printing Office.

Squire, L.R. (1987) *Memory and Brain*. New York: Oxford University Press.

Stokes, G. (1995) *Challenging Behaviour in Dementia*. Bicester: Winslow Press.

Suhi, Y. (1975) *They Fought Back*. New York: Schocken.

Summer, L. (1981) 'Guided imagery and music with the elderly.' *Music Therapy 1*, 1, 39–42.

Swartz, K., Walton, J., Crummer, G., Hantz, E. and Frisina, R. (1989) 'Does the melody linger on? Music cognition in AD.' *Seminars in Neurology 9*, 2, 152–158.

Swartz, K., Walton, J., Crummer, G., Hantz, E. and Frisina, R. (1992) 'P3 event-related potentials and performance of healthy older adults and AD subjects for music perception tasks.' *Psychomusicology 11*, 2, 96–118.

Tabloski, P., McKinnon-Howe, L. and Remington, R. (1995) 'Effects of calming music on the level of agitation in cognitively impaired nursing home residents.' *American Journal of Alzheimer's Care and Related Disorders and Research*, Jan./Feb., 10–15.

Tappen, R. (1994) 'The effect of skill training on functional abilities of nursing home residents with dementia.' *Research in Nursing and Health 17,* 159–165.

Thaut, C.H. (1999) *Melodic Intonation Therapy (MIT) Adaptations and Clinical Applications: Training in Neurologic Music Therapy.* Center for Biomedical Research in Music, Colorado State University, Fort Collins.

Thaut, M. (1999) 'Training manual for neurologic music therapy.' Unpublished manuscript, Center for Biomedical Research in Music, Colorado State University, Fort Collins.

Thomas, D., Heitman, R. and Alexander, T. (1997) 'The effects of music on bathing cooperation for residents with dementia.' *Journal of Music Therapy 34,* 246–259.

Thompson, R. (1997) 'Towards enabling communication: a study of clinical improvisation with persons with dementia.' Unpublished Master's thesis, Nordoff-Robbins Music Therapy Centre, London.

Tierney, M., Szalai, J., Snow, W. and Fisher, R. (1996) 'The prediction of Alzheimer disease: the role of patient and informant perceptions of cognitive deficits.' *Archives of Neurology 53,* 5, 423–427.

Tims, F. (1999) 'Active music making and wellness preliminary research results.' Presentation at the Music and Medicine Conference, University of Miami Medical School, Miami, April.

Tomaino, C.M. (1993a) 'Music and music therapy for the frail non-institutionalized elderly.' *Journal of Long Term Home Health Care: The PRIDE Institute Journal 13,* 2, 24–27.

Tomaino, C.M. (1993b) 'Music and the limbic system.' In F.J. Bejjani (ed) *Current Research in Arts Medicine.* Chicago: A Cappella Books.

Tomaino, C.M. (1996) 'The influence of music on memory in patients with dementia.' Final research findings NYDOH grant. Unpublished.

Tomaino, C.M. (1999) 'Music on their minds: a qualitative study of the effects of using familiar music to stimulate preserved memory function in persons with dementia.' Unpublished doctoral dissertation. New York University, New York.

Torrens, R.R. (1995) 'Hospice programmes.' *Cancer Treatment 79,* 286–292.

Tyson, J. (1989) 'Meeting the needs of dementia.' *Nursing Elders 1,* 5, 18–19.

Usita, P., Hyman, I. and Herman, K. (1998) 'Narrative intentions: listening to life stories in Alzheimer's disease.' *Journal of Aging Studies 12,* 2, 185–197.

VanderArk, S., Newman, I. and Bell, S. (1983) 'The effects of music participation on quality of life of the elderly.' *Music Therapy 3,* 1, 71–81.

Vasterling, J., Seltzer, B., Carpenter, B. and Thompson, K. (1997) 'Unawareness of social interaction and emotional control deficits in Alzheimer's disease.' *Aging Neuropsychology and Cognition 4,* 4, 280–289.

Veeh, H. Harp maker. Ochsenfürtenstr. 32, 97258 Guelchsheim.

Victoroff, J., Mack, W.J. and Nielson, K.A. (1998) 'Psychiatric complications of dementia: impact on caregivers.' *Dementia and Geriatric Cognitive Disorders 9,* 1, 50–56.

Wagner, M. and Hannon, R. (1981) 'Hemispheric asymmetries in faculty and student musicians and nonmusicians during melody recognition tasks.' *Brain and Language 13,* 379–388.

Walton, J., Frisina, R., Swartz, K., Hantz, E. and Crummer, G. (1988) 'Neural basis for music cognition: future directions and biomedical implications.' *Psychomusicology 7*, 2, 127–138.

Webster's New Encyclopedic Dictionary (1993) New York: Black Dog and Leventhal.

Werner, P., Cohen-Mansfield, J., Braun, J. and Marx, M.S. (1989) 'Physical restraints and agitation in nursing home residents.' *Journal of the American Geriatrics Society 37*, 12, 1122–1126.

Wheeler, B. (1988) 'An analysis of the literature from selected music therapy journals.' *Music Therapy Perspectives 5*, 94–101.

Whitcomb, J. (1994) '"I would weave a song for you": therapeutic music and milieu for dementia residents.' *Activities, Adaptation and Aging 18*, 2, 57–74.

White, D. and Murphy, C. (1998) 'Working memory for nonverbal auditory information in dementia of the Alzheimer type.' *Archives of Clinical Neuropsychology 13*, 4, 339–347.

Winnicott. D.W. (1971) *Playing and Reality*. London: Routledge.

Winograd, C. (1995a) 'Assessment of geriatric patients.' In D. Dale and D. Federman (eds) *Scientific American Medicine* (Section 8, Part 8, pp.1–6). New York: Scientific American.

Winograd, C. (1995b) 'Rehabilitation of geriatric patients.' In D. Dale and D. Federman (eds) *Scientific American Medicine* (Section 8, Part 10, pp.1–6). New York: Scientific American.

Wosein, M-G. (1986) *Sacred Dance*. London: Thames and Hudson.

Wylie, M.E. (1990) 'A comparison of the effects of old familiar songs, antique objects, historical summaries, and general questions on the reminiscence of nursing home residents.' *Journal of Music Therapy 27*, 1, 2–12.

Yalom, I. (1995) *The Theory and Practise of Group Psychotherapy*. New York: Basic Books.

Yonekura, Y. (1998) 'The effect of singing and physical touch on changes in voice quality of individuals with a cancer diagnosis in late stage: three case studies.' Unpublished Master's thesis, University of Kansas, Lawrence.

York, E. (1994) 'The development of a quantitative music skills test for patients with Alzheimer's Disease.' *Journal of Music Therapy 31*, 4, 280–296.

The Contributors

David Aldridge has the Chair of Qualitative Research at the Faculty of Medicine at the University of Witten-Herdecke, Germany. He is the author of *Music Therapy, Research and Practice in Medicine* and editor of *Music Therapy in Palliative Care*, also published by Jessica Kingsley Publishers.

Gudrun Aldridge works at the Institute of Music Therapy at the Univeristy of Witten-Herdecke where she teaches and supervises music therapy students. Her clinical practice is at the Institute and a nearby general hospital where she works predominantly with psychosomatic patients. She also works with breast cancer patients, chronic bowel disease patients and those suffering from Alzheimer's disease.

Melissa Brotons has worked and published extensively in the field of music therapy and dementia. She is currently based in Barcelona, Spain where she works in the Center Clinic de Musicoterapia and the University Ramon Llull.

Alicia Ann Clair is a professor, director of music therapy and research associate in gerontology at the University of Kansas, a research associate at the Colmery-O'Neil Veterans Affairs Medical Center, Topeka and a past president of the American Music Therapy Association. As a clinical researcher and practitioner, she has published widely and has consulted in the US, Canada, Denmark, Japan and Korea.

Trisha Kotai-Ewers has worked in a number of settings recoding the words of people with dementia to provide insight into the subjective experience of dementia. Originally trained as a linguist, she is currently researching a PhD at Murdich University.

Fraser Simpson is a UK state registered mucic therapist and works for East London and The City Mental Health NHS Trust within the Mental Healthcare for Older People team. He also works with children and young adults at the Nordoff–Robbins Music Therapy Centre, London.

Concetta M. Tomaino is the Director of Music Therapy at the Institute for Music and Neurologic Function at Beth Abraham Health Services where she has worked for the last twenty years. She has lectured on music therapy in Australia, South Africa, Italy and Canada and is a past president of the American Association for Music Therapy.

Annemiek Vink is a psychologist and works as a music therapy teacher at the Hogeschool Enschede, Netherlands. She is currently researching the effect of music therapy with the demented elderly for her PhD under the supervision of Prof. Dr. J.P.J. Slaets (University of Groningen, Netherlands) and Prof. Dr. David Aldridge.

Marion Violets is a senior registered dance movement therapist, working as part of a mental health team for older people in the NHS and running pilot projects in the community. She is also in private practice and gives workshops and training in therapeutic movement and dance.

Susan Weber is lecturer in music therapy at Ludwigs Maximilian University, music therapist at the Johannes Hospiz d. Barmherzigen Brüder and psychologist and music therapist at Klinikum der Universität München Grosshadern, Germany.

Subject Index

ability and emotional context
26–7
acceptance and grief 132,
134, 136
acquired brain damage 128
activation 132
active music therapy with
geriatric residents 131–5,
137, 139–40
AD *see* Alzheimer's disease
Agitation Behaviour Scale
113
agitation in elderly people
and potential benefit of
music therapy 102–18
agitation related behaviours
in dementia 103
during bathing 57, 109–10
during mealtimes 57,
110–12
effect of active music
therapy on feelings of
agitation 113
effect of individualized
music on feeling of
agitation 112–13
effect of music therapy in
reducing agitation
106–7
how does music work? 117
improvement in research
designs 116–17
specific agitation-related
behaviour changes
brought about by
musical interventions
115
what causes agitation in
dementia? 104–6
agitation scores 57
aggression, regulating 134
Alkmaar, Netherlands 122
Alzheimer's disease (AD) 12,
20, 21, 23, 25, 27,
28–32, 43, 45, 47, 52,
69–70, 72, 75, 107–9,
112, 113, 116, 121, 128,
135, 136, 139, 140,
142–6, 161–3, 168, 195,
198, 213

goals in working with AD
patients 136
and related disorders *see*
ADRD
ADRD (Alzheimer's disease
and related disorders) 34,
38, 43–7, 49–58, 61–2
American Music Therapy
Association (AMTA) 120
analogous process model 125,
126
anecdotal approaches 36–42
anecdotes as scientific stories
18–20
'Angels Wings' (Hogan,
poem) viii
Annie (elderly, dementia) 74
anxiety, regulating 134
apraxia 142
aphasia 141–2, 161
Arts in Psychotherapy 124
arts programmes, benefits for
ADRD of 38
assessment, MT 40, 46
attachment anxieties 219
attending skills 37
attention
constant requests for 103
span 163
Australia 63–80
autonomy and self-esteem
132

bathing
agitation behaviours during
57, 109–10
BCRS (Brief Cognitive
Rating Scale) 47
behaviouristic music therapy
125, 126
behaviour management 22,
36, 39, 40, 41, 42, 55–8
behaviour problems 57
'Being Myself' (May) 71
Bennett, Tony 207
'Besame Mucho' 207
biting 103
'Blue Moon' (song) 179–80
Book of Life and Death 76
Bosnia 214
Bradford Dementia Research
Group 64
brain
activity 38
mapping 39, 44
Brennan, Tim (55,
Alzheimer's) 69, 71

Brief Cognitive Rating Scale
see BCRS
Britain 120, 189, 214
Browne, Richard 85

Cagney, James 200
Canada 120, 214, 215
Canadian Association for
Music Therapy (CAMT)
120
caregivers
loneliness and self-esteem
of 39
participation socialization
and 41
and patients 23–5
programmes for 52–3
Carmen (87, dementia)
206–8
Center for Biomedical
Research in Music at
Colorado State University
98
change 20
chaplains 59
Charlie (elderly, dementia)
78–9
Christmas 208
circle work 214–17, 219,
223
classical music 130, 133, 189
clinical studies 36–42, 46,
50, 53, 55, 57
clinical benefits of musical
therapy 22
clinical changes 160–1
Clive (elderly, dementia) 75
cognitive functioning 55
cognitive music functioning
41
cognitive skills 36, 37, 39,
41, 42, 55, 57
Cohen, Dr Nicki 99
Cohen-Mansfield Agitation
Inventory 56, 103, 110,
112
coherence, temporal 28–9
coherent body and subjective
now 17–18
comfort 134
communication 32, 53
communication
establishing 132
improving 134
personal 22
social 22
stimulating 132

Author Index

Lightning Source UK Ltd.
Milton Keynes UK
09 June 2010

155261UK00003BA/7/A